An Inquiry

into the

Propagation

of

Contagious Poisons,

by the Atmosphere;

as also

Into The Nature And Effects Of Vitiated Air, Its Forms And Sources, And Other Causes Of Pestilence;

with

Directions For Avoiding The Action Of Contagion, And Observations On Some Means For Promoting Public Health

by

S. Scott Alison, M. D.
Tranent.

"I have long thought that there is no subject on which a Physician could employ his time and ability more advantageously for the benefit of his fellow-creatures, than in the investigation of febrile Contagion, in order to ascertain the laws by which it is communicated, and by what means it may be prevented."

HAYGARTH

NATAL PUBLISHING LLC
ARS LONGA, VITA BREVIS

PREFACE.

The Author trusts that the importance and the accuracy of the facts which have been detailed in the following Work may, in some measure, counterbalance the many defects which will doubtless present themselves to the reader.

The progress of the Work has been interrupted, on innumerable occasions, by the unceasing labours incident to the life of a country medical practitioner; and though many of the facts and arguments which have been used, have long obtained the author's attentive consideration, their reduction to the present form has only now been accomplished during the short intervals which he has seized, after the fatigues of the day had been concluded.

The author relies with some confidence on that indulgence which he hopes will be extended to the work of one who contributes, for useful purposes, vithe results of his experience, derived from an intimate knowledge of the condition, habits, health and diseases of the various classes of the population of a considerable extent of country, of which his situation has put him in possession.

S. S. A.

Tranent, *March 1839*.

Contents

Part I.

Introduction.

"Les hommes sont bien malheureux! ils flottent sans cesse entre de fausses esperances et des craintes ridicules; et, au lieu de s'appuyer sur la raison, ils se font des monstres qui les intimident, ou des fantomes qui les seduisent."

Montesquieu.

The author of the following pages has been induced to lay before the public the details of an investigation into Atmospheric Contagion, from the following considerations.

1st, That there prevails among the public, and especially among the relatives of the sick, much unnecessary alarm on that subject.

2d, That much injury is inflicted upon the poor patient, who is often made to suffer great and cruel privations, from the neglect and desertion of friends in a state of panic.

3d, That a great obstacle to the progress of Medical Science, is raised up by the belief in the existence of Atmospheric Contagion.

4th, That there exists relative to that subject, much confusion, from the misapplication of terms.

He has thought that these are important grievances, and that a little labour would go far to remove them. He is satisfied, from the investigation that is shortly to be detailed, that Atmospheric Contagion has no existence; that consequently all the apprehension felt upon the subject is groundless, and that the many painful measures which the public adopt, for their security, are totally unnecessary.

On a subject, too, touching such important considerations as the dreadful panic often experienced when pestilence is ravaging; the safety and ease of mind of the public; the discharge of the most sacred offices of kindness and consolation to their sick and dying fellow-men; and the progress of medical science, he has felt that the public must take a deep interest, and that he is warranted in treating it in a style fitted for popular perusal.

It must be granted that the British nation, whose sympathy is not confined among themselves, but exists for the various tribes of the human race, civilized and savage, must willingly lend an ear to an argument, whose object is, to shew that their own safety from pestilence, does not require them to be placed in the painful and cruel position, of withholding their aid from a suffering and helpless fellow-creature; of disregarding the cries and the imploring and eloquent looks of the dying; of forsaking the sick-bed of a father or a brother, denying the tender and unpurchaseable offices of friendship, and of ruthlessly breaking asunder the sacred bonds with which God has wisely and indulgently joined us.

They, whose hearts are open to the appeal of the forlorn slave, must be gratified to hear that they may perform the offices of humanity to their sick relatives and friends, without, as has hitherto been thought, subjecting themselves to the almost certain invasion of disease; that they may watch the last moments of an expiring friend, minister to his latest wants, and have the melancholy gratification of standing by him, when about to make the last and most awful change that can overtake him.

It is expected that it will be shewn, that the sick-room is at all times free of the poison with which it has been believed to be contaminated, and that the atmosphere there, if attention is paid to ventilation, &c. is almost as wholesome as that out of doors.

The air which the sick respire does become impure, but not on ordinary occasions in a manner different, or with a greater virulence, than is observed in the case of air in a small and close apartment, respired by many persons closely huddled together.

The history of sick chambers presents no instance more dreadful than that of the Black Hole of Calcutta, where so many perished of corrupted or vitiated air.

The subject of infectious air touches directly upon the most important interests of mankind, concerns intimately their safety, the duties of man to man, and even the very affections of the heart.

As the subject at present stands, the public is awkwardly situated; believing that they must either endanger their health, even their lives, or allow their friends and relatives to perish unassisted.

The author thinks he is under no obligation to apologize for attempting to shew, that the public may at once perform all the charities of life to the sick, and avoid the action of a virulent poison. There can be none necessary, and he even hopes that his inquiry may tend to obtain for many, who are yet to be the victims of pestilence, that succour from hands they love, which, alas! has been withheld from thousands.

It has not been usual to write speculative medical opinions in a popular style, but the author is of opinion that an inquiry bearing on matters so important, should be made known to those whom it most concerns, certainly, the people; and he is convinced, that in a simple case of evidence such as this, that they are qualified to decide, provided there is a full and impartial leading of facts on both sides, and there be absence of all technical terms and purely professional phrases. The discussion will be conducted on plain and obvious principles, so that the merits of the question may be appreciated, at once, by them and the profession.

The public is already informed of much that relates to the animal economy in health, through the assistance of many admirable works which have been published within the last few years, and it is not unfair to suppose that they may be interested in hearing, and likewise capable of understanding, a case relative to disease.

The community is aware that Medicine is not now the subtle, hidden, affectedly mysterious art, it was at no very remote date; and that its present enlightened professors now seek not the assistance of darkness, of silence, to disguise their ignorance and questionable views, or to heighten the impression of the skill and cunning of their order.

Its study is now conducted openly, and its foundation, happily, is laid upon principles established in nature that are as well known to the unprofessional as to the professional man.

There is no wish to disguise matters from the public, and, were it attempted, it could not possibly succeed.

The utmost care will be observed to lay the evidence impartially down, plainly, and divested of technical phraseology; and, satisfied of the general ability of the public to judge, the author will await their decision with as much anxiety as that of the medical world.

It will afford the writer the return he most values, if, by his means, less anxiety and apprehension are felt in future among the public on occasions of disease; if those acting under a sense of duty are enabled to discharge their humane offices with less feeling of danger; if the patient remain unoppressed with alarm for the dear ministering friends around him; if even one sufferer be spared the anguish of bearing wants unanswered, and if in his last hours he is spared the bitterness of soul he must experience, when deserted by those to whom, through life, he looked for comfort and support.

The author has also been induced to publish his views upon vitiated air, its nature, sources and effects, with directions for its prevention, avoidance, and correction. Vitiated air has been confounded with atmospheric contagion, has performed the greater part of the work of death attributed to that agency, or supposed agency, and it has been it that has been affected and controlled, when both non-professional people and the medical world thought systems of quarantine, isolation, gens des cordons, (contagion police,) and fumigations, were effecting the objects for which they were established.

The immediate objects of these counteracting agents, the destruction of contagion and contagious atmosphere, &c., could not be effected, since, at least, the latter does not exist: but fortunately, though they could not effect the objects immediately proposed, the ultimate ends have been served, by their acting on many occasions upon the efficient causes of disease, viz. vitiated air.

They were useful after the fashion of the medicine and charms in olden times, used for the expulsion of evil spirits, devils, and the like, which, by their natural action upon the functions of the body, corrected derangements which were mistaken for the operations of these imaginary beings. The Author has pointed out other causes of pestilence, and has given some directions for their prevention, and for the preservation of health.

Chapter I.

Prevalence of Doctrine of Atmospheric Contagion, Injury to Patient, Attendants and Visitors

Atmospheric contagion, to which public attention is directed, has been regarded for many ages as the cause of a great proportion of the pestilence incident to the human race; and, at the present day, most of the diseases which are wont to be widely spread, and to be very mortal, are usually considered as depending on that agent, both by the unprofessional and the medical world: indeed, so extended has been thought its sphere of action, that it is suspected to be operating in almost every case that occurs, of those diseases which usually attack many at the same time; and, in nearly every instance, its existence is positively inferred, where previous cases can be shewn to have been prevailing, though at the distance of several miles.

It is a fact familiar to many, that, on the occasion of the late prevalence of Cholera Morbus in the years 1831 and 1832, that infection, through the medium of the air, was considered the most common cause of the propagation of that scourge; and every mother is taught to regard every case of scarlet fever, common fever, hooping-cough, and many such disorders, as a very centre of infectious air that possesses qualities subversive of the health of her children.

Ordinary conversation, too, marks well the common belief in the positive injury that agent inflicts. In general, it seems a matter quite out of the question to suppose, that the patient may have got his sickness from the operation of other and distinct causes, as is sufficiently evident from such common questions as these, "Had he visited any person ill of the same complaint?"—"Where, and from whom, did he get the infection?" and likewise from the ordinary replies, "He got it from a friend, at whose house he called to inquire after his health,"—"He caught it when passing through a street in which a person lay ill of the same distemper." Such inquiries and replies are made not only by the public, but by the medical profession also, who are, in general, sufficiently satisfied if such answers and solutions as those above be given. Were it necessary to say more to prove the important position infection holds as a cause of disease, and as the chief instrument of its propagation, references might be made to thousands of instances, narrated, too, on medical authority, where whole visitations of pestilence have been attributed to its operation, and volumes might be filled with the most skilful artifices, devised, and actually carried into execution, to deprive the air of its invisible poison; but these steps are deemed unnecessary here.

The belief in the doctrine of atmospheric contagion is hurtful to the patient by its direct influence on his mind, and the gratification of his wishes.

The patient laid on the bed of sickness, having many wants and occasions for a thousand little offices, but being unable to assist himself, generally desires, and, where apprehension does not cause desertion, obtains the aid of good and gentle friends, whose very presence affords a gratification to the sufferer which none can sufficiently value, who have not, like him, felt its blessings. Their assistance and constant presence is absolutely necessary to supply his several wants, and to render a situation, often painful, and ever irksome, less acutely so.

But not more necessary is such assistance to the mitigation of the sufferings of the body, and the soothing, the calming of a fevered mind, than is it urgently wished for, and longed for by the patient, to whom even the momentary absence of the ministering being from his bedside is frequently the cause of much mental agitation and of pain.

But where, as we have often seen, the patient has still his senses left, and dearly loves the objects around him, what must be the amount of that bitterness of mental struggle going on in his breast, alternately heaving with desire for their presence as his greatest comfort, and with the alarm every amiable being must feel, lest those most dear to him should fall the victims of their tenderness, and be cut down themselves, in their holy endeavours to relieve his sufferings?

The apprehensions of the patient lest those kind and beloved friends ministering to his wants, and nobly incurring on his account all the risk of a dangerous situation, should unhappily derive from him, through the medium of Atmospheric Contagion, the same disease,—are calculated to produce a state of excitement highly injurious and directly opposed to that calm and cheerful state of mind so favourable to his recovery. But these apprehensions are often changed for the dreadful reality, and no little mental suffering has been produced, and no trifling obstacle to the convalescence of a patient has been raised up, by the intimation that a dear friend has caught the pestilence from him, and has in consequence been deprived of life.

The belief in the doctrine of Atmospheric Contagion is hurtful also to the friends and attendants of the patient—by its naturally conveying the impression that he is a centre of a poisonous agent, whose immediate tendency is to propagate the distemper and diffuse itself through the atmosphere, extending to it, its deleterious attributes, to be felt by all who respire it.

The poison is said to diffuse itself in the air of the apartment; hence it is believed, that entering into the apartment is tantamount to destruction, or at least, is nothing less than exposure to an influence of the most virulent and deadly quality.

It does not at the time signify to the attendants, the evidence on which the doctrine rests. It is believed, and that is enough to cause the most baneful effects upon the spirits, to inspire the worst apprehensions, and has also, as is well known, produced those very effects they had feared from its operation, has caused the increase of disease, nay, death itself, and that not on one occasion only, but on many.

The most common causes of Pestilence, Plague, Putrid and low Fevers, and Cholera, are mostly of a depressing nature, and, usually, the more they partake of that character, they are the more effectual in their operation. Famine is chiefly favourable to the sickness which is usually coincident with it, from the depressed and feeble state of body it produces; and an impure atmosphere is deleterious, chiefly from its allowing the body to become less energetic, by withholding that vigour and elasticity which the respiration of pure air imparts to the system at large, and thence to the mind.

These are powerful depressing causes, but not more so than fear, especially that kind that is deep and lasts long. Moral philosophers rank Fear as one of the most depressing passions, and its characteristics with the artist are paleness, contraction of the features, the best and surest indication of a weakened circulation (of blood) and diminution of vital power. The first are well aware of the hurtful influence it imparts to the whole body, and narrate instances, on excellent authority, where death, even immediate death, has been the consequence, where the brain has had its functions impaired, and thus imbecility induced; so that in short, they are accustomed to regard it as one of the most powerful agents, applied both to the mind and body.

The Medical Philosopher, too, has frequent occasion to mark the great depression of the powers of the body, the imperfect discharge of its functions, and the general exhaustion consequent upon the long continued operation of apprehension.

Be the apprehension of whatever nature, it is always detrimental—in a ratio too, proportionate to its intensity, and its other contingent circumstances. In the lesser degrees, it causes indigestion, flatus, loss of appetite, headach, and often general restlessness, with feelings of great discomfort.

It is found operating with great force, whether it arise from apprehension of damnation in respect to a future state, of ruin in a pecuniary point of view, or perhaps from what is most immediate and striking in its effects, of catching the infection of pestilential disease, which is the point with which we have most to do.

We have known many persons much affected with the fear of taking infection, and allowing this to prey upon their spirits, who were among the first attacked with pestilence; and if any weight is to be given to our knowledge of the probable causes of disease, there is great reason for concluding that those persons were the victims of their very fears, more than of any other causes of a prejudicial character. It is often impossible, with complete justice, to say decidedly that any one influence has been the exclusive cause of disease, when there is room to think there are, or may be many ready to operate; but, in many instances, the relation has been so immediate, and so striking between the known presence of depressing apprehension, and the supervention of sickness, that there is no room left to doubt the propriety of placing them in the relation of cause and effect. It must be familiar to many, quite a common occurrence, and one of which we heard constantly during the ravages of Cholera a few years ago, that persons took that disease from mere fright, and of the attack having been very much encouraged by its operation among the attendants, and more especially of those believing in the existence of the infectious nature of the disease.

These facts, it is thought, will prove that the doctrine of Atmospheric Contagion is calculated to excite much apprehension among the attendants and visitors of one sick of pestilence, and to shew in what manner that very apprehension is disposed to produce disease.

The attendant or visitor persuaded of the atmospherically contagious character of the disease, must possess considerable fortitude to venture at all into the presence of the patient, and even when once there, he must possess more than common hardihood, who does not feel more or less depressed with apprehension for that potent, and not the less imposing agent, because invisible, which, like a drawn sword, hangs over him, and threatens his existence.

By the belief in the doctrine of Atmospheric Contagion, the attendant not only becomes, in general, exposed to one of the most common and efficient causes of disease, viz. fear, but his offices are performed more as a duty than as a gratification, which it is to a well disposed mind, where no extraordinary danger is encountered, and he is thus forced to make a sacrifice of his feelings, and the valued assurance of security to a rigid sense of duty; but however much such conduct may agree with morals, it is detrimental to health.

It is hurtful also to the patient, from its influencing so far those, who, by relationship, by previous terms of friendship, and by duty, are bound, by every moral obligation, to assist him, now helpless, sick, and perhaps expiring,—as to forget their most sacred duties as to make them disregard his forlorn situation, and indeed to induce them to fly from and desert him; thus sacrificing every good principle and wholesome consideration, (as they erroneously think) to make their own lives the more secure.

Such contingencies are of frequent occurrence; and the result is, that many unhappy persons are left to perish, their thirst unslaked, their latest requests unheard, and their last moments unwitnessed. Parents have been known to forsake their children, and the offspring their parents, whom, at all hazards, they were bound to serve,—by every holy affection, to assist the more diligently, the more they were pressed with adversity.

But alas! the affections, the instincts of Nature, the dictates of gratitude, have been thrown aside, and every thing fair and holy in the human soul has been foully stained, in the almost universal wreck, attendant on the course of pestilence.

The history of the cholera visitation affords many examples of perishing persons deserted and left to the mercy of a cruel scourge; and we are familiar with many instances which have come under our own charge, where it has been found impossible to procure the attendance of relations, or even the mercenary aid of hirelings, although extraordinary remuneration has been offered.

Last winter, the father and mother of a family were seized with fever, and their sole attendants were their infant children. There were several relatives of the family not far off, but none, not even one, could be persuaded to lend assistance. Their neighbours refused to hold any communication; and, notwithstanding repeated and continued attempts by the Author to induce those who make it their business to wait upon the sick, the family had to struggle on, without the least attention being paid, saving by the almost useless children, to their wants, to cleanliness, and to the administration of the remedies.

It was truly a deplorable scene, such as made the Author reprobate that cowardly desertion, and regret the operation of a doctrine so baneful, and moreover so groundless. Yet we know not whether to blame most the people or the doctrine. Did those see the scenes, the distress and cruelty inflicted through the operation of infectious air, who believe in it, and preach its avoidance; surely, did they possess one spark of humanity, it could not fail to manifest itself, by causing them to institute, or at least to listen to, an inquiry touching its evidence.

The medical attendants are not free from the hurtful operation of this doctrine. If believers in infectious air, they are under a feeling of apprehension which, perhaps with some, may not be strongly felt, on account of the frequency of impunity from exposure; but with many it is strongly felt, and influences their attendance on the sick, their communication with them, and their own comfort and feeling of security.

Many instances are known—they are of very frequent occurrence—where the physician, from apprehension, has failed to pay so many visits as were necessary, or to remain with his patient sufficiently long to ascertain his situation, and watch well the progress of the case. Cases are known where patients have been looked at by their advisers, stationed at the door, where it was impossible to ascertain the expression of the countenance, the condition of the tongue, the state of the skin, not to say any thing of that of the pulse.

We are acquainted with instances in which medical men have so acted under the apprehension of taking infection, and where, too, they have not felt they were doing any thing reprehensible, as was sufficiently evident from the fact, that they themselves were the informants.

These facts prove that injury has been done to the patient from insufficient care; and cases are not wanting, where medical men themselves have taken disease, where the circumstances of the case warranted the belief that fear was the chief, if not the only cause. Many very cunningly-devised plans have been recommended for the adoption of the physicians visiting patients labouring under infectious diseases, such as standing in a current of air passing between windows, or doors and windows,—keeping a handkerchief applied to the mouth and nose, washing the mouth with water, &c. These are sometimes adopted, yet there is room to think that, where a man of merely ordinary fortitude supposes that he inspires an atmosphere holding in solution a very virulent, nay deadly poison, that he will be anxious to make his visit as short as possible, even though the preventives above mentioned be religiously adopted.

Several of the cases of death among medical men, which have been unhesitatingly attributed to infectious air, the Author is convinced, from his knowledge of particular circumstances, and from the known tendency of fear, have arisen from depression, in consequence of that passion.

The prejudicial operation of the doctrine of infectious air has been proved in reference to the patient himself, *1st*, From his apprehension for the safety of others ministering to him; *2d*, From the neglect and desertion of friends and others; *3d*, From the insufficient medical treatment which his case frequently obtains.

It has been proved in reference to friends and attendants, who are often in consequence in a state of apprehension, favouring the invasion of disease; and in relation to the first, who are made to regard one of the most delightful offices as a duty of imminent peril.

It is hurtful both to patient and friend, by forbidding that intercourse which, but for the danger in question, would be so delightful and consoling to both.

It tends to the commission of crimes of no trifling character, the desertion of kindred and of friends, the hardening and debasing of the heart, and the general corruption of the finest sentiments that bind and ornament society.

It has led to deeds not the least dark in the page of human history.

It takes much from the efficiency of medicine, and has been the frequent cause of much evil to its professors.

For all those reasons, it is an important subject, and demands patient investigation.

Surely a case has been made out to shew how important are its effects, and how much evil might be avoided were it proven, as is proposed to be done, that Atmospheric Contagion has no existence. That is all, that is desired to be shewn from what precedes, and we would on no account wish the amount of mischief it inflicts to be thought as put forward as an argument against its entity, which would be absurd.

Chapter II

Medicine Retarded—Forms of Contagion

The progress of medical science has been much impeded by the operation of the doctrine of atmospheric contagion. From the earliest periods the practitioners of medicine have been in the habit of attributing a very great proportion of the worst forms of disease to that agent; and the consequence has been that little attention has been paid to the investigation of the most difficult, and not the least important department, that of the efficient and ordinary causes of disease.

It was almost a necessary consequence of the possession of such an instrument, ready on all occasions, to solve the problems offered by the occurrences of disease, that no inquiry would be made into those circumstances by which might be detected those influences that conduce to its production. There was ever at hand an agent whose existence all were alike ready to concede, which was amply sufficient to explain the origin and propagation of pestilence.

That being the case, medical men had no inducement to make investigations, and from one generation to another they have gone on in the old way, attributing much to that agency, and leaving uninquired into, with few exceptions, the actual springs of diseased action.

Until very lately little was known of the relation between disease and such important matters as these,—the state of the atmosphere, the severities of the weather, and its other contingent circumstances, the quality of the food and drink, clothing, habits, climate, and the like.

These most important matters received very little consideration, and although much has lately been done to shew their influence in the origin and propagation of disease; yet they are not regarded as so efficient in that respect as they ought to be, and the reason of it is, that the common application of atmospheric contagion to the explanation of the problem, by the vast majority of medical practitioners, puts a stop to the scrutiny which would detect their relation. The fact undoubtedly is, that, in respect to some diseases, little is known, among those intrusted with their treatment, of their causes. This situation of affairs is dangerous, and were physicians to adopt the extravagant measures, which the doctrine of atmospheric contagion suggests, there is a risk that, armed with weapons of so powerful a nature as our medicines are, and moreover, applied to so delicate and nicely strung a machine as the human body, their interference might become downright tampering, and dangerous in the extreme.

But the blame does not lie so much with the present generation of practitioners. It is more the fault of the science than of its present professors.

That doctrine has been taught them, as on established and well authenticated principle. They have too readily confided in the accuracy of their predecessors, and taken for ascertained, that which was only supposititious. Still the public injury is the same, be that as it may; and would the profession perform efficiently its important duties, and deserve that confidence so necessary for the full operation of the art, they would, without delay, inquire into the merits of this case, and turn to the investigation of the causes of disease, the many facts and principles, revealed by the late rapid progress of the sciences.

For the judicious and efficient treatment of disease, a knowledge of its causes is necessary. The disorders being ascertained, the first consideration in reference to the treatment is the cause or causes, and according as the information partakes of certainty or uncertainty, so the propriety of the measures is sure or doubtful.

Without a knowledge of the causes, sure or probable, our efforts are, in some cases, like random blows made in the dark, they may or may not strike the object. It is in general only when the causes are known, more or less, particularly, that medical treatment can be said to rest on a sure and philosophical basis, and to promise the full amount of benefit the art can afford.

For many years the investigation of Atmospheric

Contagion has occupied the Author, anxious only to ascertain its actual merits, and to be guided by the result, free of prejudice or bias.

The result has been, that from the actual, constant, and minute observation of disease, from an enlarged inquiry into the circumstances coincident therewith, of the pestilential character of many agencies, and a careful comparison with every agent or form in nature with which we are acquainted, bearing any resemblance to what Atmospheric Contagion must be, if it have an existence at all; that where other hurtful influences are operating, Atmospheric Contagion is needlessly called in to account for their effects, and that it (*i. e.* Atmospheric Contagion) has no existence, properly considered, in the light of an atmosphere holding in solution a specific contagious poison.

Before commencing the argument, it is proposed to notice shortly its history, and the opinions held at this day respecting its nature and qualities.

But as these opinions are very various and conflicting, and as, moreover, from the general confusion of terms, the reader will almost unavoidably become perplexed and unable to understand the merits of the case as treated here or by others, the Author proposes to explain, before going further, what is meant or ought to be meant by contagion, and by contagious air. He is not aware that any plain and uniform method or arrangement of the principles in question is in common use, though some physicians, as will appear in the historical sketch that is to follow, have reduced contagion to two or three distinct kinds, and thus divested the subject of much of its perplexing clashing of terms. They have given fixed meanings to some terms formerly used by all, and even at present by most, with too great latitude.

We will consider, *1st*, Contagion.

That term is, and with propriety may be, used to denote that property, which matter eliminated in a body suffering under disease, has of producing the same disease when applied to another in a state of health, as the matter of small-pox.

Contagion is also used, and will be employed here, to denote the matter itself which we have just defined.

Thus it appears that contagion is used to signify both the property of the matter and the matter itself. This should be understood, as confusion may lead to great misconception. In the same way, the term "heat" is used to denote caloric itself, and also its property.

Contagion, signifying the matter itself, is said to act in different shapes, but here medical men divide. According to those on whose authority most reliance is to be placed, they are the following—three in number:—

1st, By the direct application to the body of palpable contagious matter.

2dly, By the application to the body of clothes, and the like, impregnated with contagious matter.

3dly, By the application to the body of air holding in solution, contagious matter.

To contagion acting in the first-mentioned manner, has almost universally been applied the title, by distinction, Contagion, or immediate contagion; but in order to promote perspicuity, we shall call it Contactual or Palpable Contagion.

To contagion acting in the second-mentioned manner, has been applied the term Fomites (impregnated clothes), but we shall call it Fomitic Contagion.

To contagion acting in the third-mentioned manner, many terms have been applied indiscriminately, Contagion, Infection, Contagious Miasm, Infectious Air, &c. &c.; but to preserve distinctness, and to shew its relation to the other modes, we shall apply to it the title Atmospheric Contagion.

With Atmospheric Contagion, the third mode in which contagion acts, has been confounded by many, air holding in solution, or having commingled with it, gases or impurities, not producing exclusively one disease, as contagious matter does; but productive of deranged health—or at least hurtful to life.

Air thus tainted, has also been called Contagious, Infectious, &c. &c.; but as it is widely different, for the reason mentioned, they should not be confounded; and in order to prevent any accidental confusion, we shall term it vitiated, or, simply, impure air.

There is yet another pestiferous principle called Marsh Miasm, which has sometimes, but less frequently, been confounded with the third mode in which contagion acts, viz. atmospheric contagion. They are very different: the former is confined to marshy lands, and produces exclusively disease of an intermittent character.

Of the first mode in which contagion is said to act, contactual or palpable contagion, there is the most positive proof. That is a settled point capable of demonstration.

Of the second, viz. fomitic contagion, there seems to be no good room to doubt. It is consistent with our knowledge, on points of a like nature, to admit the possibility of its existence; and there is evidence of pretty good character, that contagion does act in that shape, though we are disposed to think that it is not the cause of pestilence so often as is generally understood.

It is to the third mode, viz. atmospheric contagion, that we object. We question its existence for these reasons, *first*, That in the whole course of its history, it fails to supply us with sufficient evidence thereof; *secondly*, That its supposed career is not marked with the same uniformity of effect, and constancy of character, cognisable among other powerful agents, but appears rather to be regulated by no fixed laws; *thirdly*, That the phenomena of disease do not go to shew that it is dependent on atmospheric contagion, the occurrence and dissemination of which, moreover, it could not explain.

We are further disposed to deny its existence at all, for this reason, that its admission is opposed to the testimony of direct observation and of experiments instituted for the purpose.

CHAPTER III

Historical Sketch

In the Old Testament, frequent allusion is made to contagion, particularly in Leviticus, where directions are given for the expurgation, from the system, of that principle; for the isolation of persons possessed of it; and the cleansing of garments therewith infected.

The earliest Grecian historians make reference to it, and Thucydides, in his History of the Plague, attributes some occurrences in its career, to the operation of that principle.

Dr Winterbottom[1] writes thus, of an ancient physician—"Aratæus says, that the miserable patients (those ill of Elephantiasis), were banished into deserts, or to the top of mountains, where the kindness of their friends occasionally attended their distresses; though perhaps they were more frequently deserted."

Cælius Aurelianus, a noted physician, says—"Some advise that a person labouring under this disease, should be turned out of town, if a stranger, or if an inhabitant, be banished to some distant part; others advise the patient to be totally abandoned."

These expressions relate to contagion generally.

Atmospheric contagion is not specified, though perhaps even then, it may have been thought to exist.

As already said, later physicians thought that contagious diseases were propagated in three different ways, *1st*, by actual contact with the matter or virus itself; *2dly*, by fomites, or by contact with clothes tainted with it; and, *3dly*, by infection, or by air holding it in solution.

But it is to contagion, as diffused through the air, that the observations that are to follow are directed. So we shall, for the present at least, dismiss the other two modes of its action,

[1] Dr Winterbottom on Sierra Leone.

that by contact, and that by fomites or tainted clothes, with the expression of our belief in their existence, as modes of the propagation of disease.

In 1777, Dr Haygarth, an English physician, began to investigate the laws that regulate the action of contagious poisons, and for the first time they obtained a scientific examination, and became the subject of experiment, if, perhaps, are excepted the labours of Lind, whose observations appeared about the same time.

Dr Haygarth believed in the propagation of disease through the direct application of contagious matter, such, for instance, as that of small-pox; but of this none have expressed any doubt worthy of notice; for the fact is well known, and often witnessed, by inoculation for small-pox and cow-pox.

At the time at which Dr Haygarth wrote, very vague and extravagant notions were held on the subject of contagious poisons diffused in the air—of air holding in solution contagious poison, or, as we have determined to call it—Atmospheric Contagion.

It was believed to extend itself to great distances, and there to develope its powers.

His opinions on the subject were, at the time of their publication, quite original; and as they are such as are usually held, to this day, by most intelligent practitioners, the most important will be transcribed here.

In a letter to Dr Percival, on the prevention of infectious diseases, published in 1801, Dr H. says—"I have long thought that there is no subject on which a physician could employ his time and ability more advantageously for the benefit of his fellow-creatures, than in the investigation of febrile contagion, in order to ascertain the laws by which it is communicated, and by what means it may be prevented. It is well known to be the cause of very extensive destruction in the army, the navy, and in large towns."

"In 1777 I began to ascertain, by clinical observations, (*i. e.* observations made at the bedside of a patient,) according to what law the small-pox infection, and, in 1780 and 1781, according to what law the febrile infection, is propagated."—"I found that the pernicious effects of small-pox miasms (that is, airs or vapours) were limited to a very narrow sphere. In the open air, and in moderate cases, I discovered that the infectious distance does not exceed half a yard."—"Hence it is probable that, even when the distemper is malignant, the infectious influence extends to but a few yards from the poison."—"I soon also discovered, that the contagion of fevers was confined to a much narrower sphere."

"You will recollect, my dear friend, that at this time (1781) my attention was much engaged in the investigation of the nature of the small-pox poison. I was struck with the difference of the periods in those two maladies during which the infection remains in a latent state, that is, the interval of time which elapses between the patient's exposure to the pestilential influence and the commencement of the fever. In the typhus, this period appeared to be much longer than in small-pox."

The period between the exposure to what is considered infection, and the period of the manifestation of disease, certainly does vary in different distempers. In those in which palpable contagious poisons are produced, and where they are palpably applied to the system, the interval is known, and seldom varies; but in those where a palpable poison is not recognised, or where it is said to act exclusively through the air, it is found that the interval is sometimes short, sometimes long, and manifests none of that precision almost always observed in reference to the first class of diseases.

Dr Haygarth again says, "When the room of a patient ill of an infectious fever is spacious, airy, and clean, few or none of the most intimate attendants will catch the disease."

"Among the middle and higher ranks of society in Chester and its neighbourhood, during a period of thirty-one years, I scarcely recollect a single instance of the typhus fever being communicated to a second person, not even during the epidemics of 1783 and 1786, which excited a general alarm in that city, Fresh air and cleanliness were the only means which I employed to prevent infection. Doors and windows were kept open as far as the season, and other circumstances, would permit. Curtains were drawn to exclude the light, but not the free circulation of air. All clothes, utensils, &c. used by the patient were immersed in a vessel of cold water immediately, and, when taken out of it, carefully washed. The floors were kept clean, and vinegar was sometimes, but not always, employed to sprinkle. It was thought to be more easy to remove than to correct the poison."

Dr Haygarth deserves much credit for his judicious treatment, and by it he had the satisfaction of seeing much public good effected. His principles are yet acted upon with the very best effects; but it will be shewn, at a more advanced part of this work, that the check put to the progress of disease, was rather to be attributed to the removal of an atmosphere loaded with unwholesome emanations, than to any power those steps or measures had, of rendering innocuous, by dilution, a specific contagious poison.

Dr Haygarth continues—"The whole evidence which I have been able to collect, incontestibly leads to this very important conclusion, that febrile infection extends but to a very narrow sphere from the person.

"It appears highly improbable that the typhus infection should ever be communicated in the open air, by the common intercourse of society; because visitors, and even attendants, with very few exceptions, escape the fever, when exposed to it, in even the same chamber, if clean, airy, and spacious.

"The quantity of miasms (unwholesome or poisonous air) respired in the latter, is incomparably more than it can be in the former situation. It is not, however, intended to be asserted that such an event is impossible, if a person on purpose, or by some rare accident, were to breathe the air which immediately issues from a patient, or from clothes fully impregnated with the poison.

"During my long attention to this inquiry, not a single instance ever occurred to prove that persons liable to the small-pox could associate in the same chamber with a patient in the distemper, without receiving the infection.

"We have no certain knowledge in what manner infectious fevers are received into the body. According to the most plausible conjecture they appear to be communicated by poisonous vapours, which issue from the breath, or the insensible perspiration, or the excretions of a patient in the distemper. These miasms are probably taken into the body by the absorbents of the mouth, nostrils, lungs, stomach, or skin."

Under the able investigation of Dr Haygarth, the doctrine of infection has been deprived of much of its extravagant character. Under his examination it is found losing that widely extended range of action, and that extreme virulence, that had hitherto marked its history.

Dr Bateman, in his excellent work on contagious fever, after alluding to a prevalent opinion, that contagious poison is capable of diffusion in the air, says, "To one acquainted with the evidence which has been adduced relative to the properties of contagion, these opinions, and the terrors connected with them, appear equally unfounded and absurd, as are all creations of an over-excited imagination magnified by prejudice and alarm—for it has been proved, beyond the possibility of a doubt, by the concurrent testimony of a multitude of the ablest practitioners, who have had every opportunity of investigating the fact, and by all the experience which the establishment of fever boards and houses of recovery has afforded the means of accumulating, that no contagion whatever is communicable, even to the distance of a few feet, through the medium of the free and open atmosphere, and consequently that residence in a district where fever prevails is free from all danger. Nay, it has been further proved on the same undeniable evidence, that the house and even the apartment, occupied by the sick, may be rendered perfectly innocuous, the contagion being disarmed of its activity and virulence by dilution with pure air," &c.

Dr Bateman gives the following facts—

"All the patients admitted into the London House of Recovery are transported in a litter by two others employed by the institution, enveloped in their uncleanly and tainted apparel. Yet the porters who have been daily occupied for the last eighteen months in conveying this double source of contagion, often the distance of two or three miles, and assisting them in and out of the litter, have never received the infection.

"Neither have the washerwomen, employed during the period of my attendance, (sixteen years) on the House of Recovery, occupied almost constantly in washing the apparel brought in by the patient, as well as the bed-linen, often much soiled by their excretions, and the cloths used by the patients in the house, ever been affected with the fever."

Dr Patrick Russell, whose work on the plague is so well known, is the next writer to whose observations reference will be made. His personal observation of much contagious disease, and his high character, entitle his observations to much weight. They will amply shew, how the question before us has gained with the advancement of medical science. Some are subjoined.

"In the first place, the various and vague application of the term contagion has been the source of confusion. In foreign languages, as well as in English, it has sometimes been used for the plague itself, sometimes as synonimous with infections; sometimes for the virulent effluvia issuing from the sick, or from substances infected, and sometimes as a property common to various diseases."

He is of the decided opinion, that plague is communicated, by contact of the body, with the poison, which is properly understood by the word contagion. He says—"The second mode of contagion is by the medium of the air. The effluvia arising from the diseased, received into the ambient air, form a pestiferous atmosphere, more or less impregnated with these effluvia, as it recedes from their source. That contagion is thus communicated in the chamber of the sick, appears from persons being infected without touching the diseased body, or any thing in the room that may be supposed to harbour infection.

"To what distance the tainted atmosphere extends is not yet known, but recent facts render it probable that the effluvia, when once transmitted into the air, are soon dispersed, blended with the common mass, or otherwise suffer such alteration as render them innocuous at no great distance from their source. It is probable, also, that those effluvia arise, in an active state, to no great height in the atmosphere."

He adds, that the contagion by fomites, that is, impregnated clothes, is the most extensive in its operation; and that it spreads disease, not only in all quarters of a town, but also to remote regions. He asserts that the plague is conveyed into different streets, remote from one another, by the Jewish salesmen, and that he has known Armenian washerwomen infected by tainted linen. The infectious air of plague, according to him, when it adheres to substances not exposed to free ventilation, and closely packed, retains its vigour for along time, and in that state is transported to other countries: and he held it as proven that it retains its activity in a three months' voyage from the coast of Syria to Marseilles.

He is disposed to think that the contagion of plague, rarely remains in the system longer than ten days, and that more danger is to be apprehended from the baggage of passengers who enter into lazarettoes, than from their persons.

To Dr Joseph Adams we are indebted for an excellent treatise on animal poisons, one that is much valued for the information and clear views it contains. The following is an extract from the work in question.

"By contagion I would understand those diseases with the origin of which we are now unacquainted, but which at present can only be propagated by contact with a person, or matter from a person under similar disease. Contagious diseases, which it is now our business to consider, may be divided into chronic and acute, of the former are the itch, and several others. These are for the most part incurable by the unassisted powers of the constitution. The acute of which are the small-pox, and many other exanthemata, (these are those diseases accompanied with fever) marked with a peculiar eruption, and that attack only once, such as measles, and scarlet fever produce a critical fever, which ceases with the disease.

"The chronic may attack a person as often as he is exposed to the exciting cause, the acute, for the most part, leave the constitution no longer susceptible of their operation."

After pointing out the modes of communication of contagious diseases by contact and by fomites, he says, "Infectious diseases, on the contrary, may be traced in their origin, and do not require for their production matter similar to their effects, but may at any time be generated by crowding together the sick or wounded of any description. Of this kind are the hospital, prison, or ship-fever, camp dysentery, and some peculiarly malignant ulcers. Though these diseases, when formed, may produce their like in others, yet we can always trace their origin to causes different from their effects."

From the London Cyclopædia the following extract is taken.

"There does not appear to be any distinction commonly made between contagious and infectious diseases."

This extract proves how much confusion there exists, with the terms infectious and contagious. Here they are said to be used synonimously, and in that of Dr Bateman just quoted, a great distinction is drawn.

Such are a few of the facts connected with the history of contagion, which are most worthy of notice, in a work of this kind.

This sketch will afford some idea of the most rational views which have been, and still are, held on the subject; and of the light in which it is at present regarded by the medical world.

It is feared that the extracts which have been given, may appear too copious, but it has been thought highly proper, that the opinions of those justly considered, the greatest authorities on the subject, should be given: and that they might not be misunderstood, they have been, for the most part, presented verbatim.

CHAPTER IV

The Absence of Sufficient Evidence of The Existence of Atmospheric Contagion

Ponderable bodies are endowed with common or general properties, and likewise with particular or secondary properties.

Magendie

The properties of atmospheric contagion, under its various titles, have been noted in the preceding chapter. They have been attributed to it, by the most eminent writers on the subject, and are such as are assented to, by most medical men of the present day.

Its origin, the sphere of its activity, and the means by which it may be destroyed or neutralized, have there been alluded to. In the extracts given, and in the current medical literature of the present time, it is spoken of, as an agent of whose existence there is the utmost assurance.

The reader who has not already thought upon the subject for himself, but has, as is almost universally done, in reference to this agent, taken the whole case, as one fully ascertained, and settled upon fixed principles, will doubtless be surprised to hear, that it is the decided opinion of a member of the medical profession, that the doctrine of atmospheric contagion presents no sufficient evidence of its truth; that he is in possession of facts connected with the occurrence of disease, which render it probable, that other and efficient causes of disease have been thrown aside, to make room for that agency, and that he is convinced, from the results of experiments on contagious poisons, and from a minute inquiry into their nature, that it (that is, atmospheric contagion) does not exist. Perhaps he should regret that he has not been able to see the question in the same light as his brethren. He has felt unwilling to espouse singular opinions;

he has therefore been patient in the inquiry, and it has been only from the consideration, that a great medical truth was concerned, that the progress of the science might possibly, thereby, be promoted, and that the comfort of the patient, and the ease of mind, of the public, might be advanced, that he has been induced to lay his opinions before the world.

Regarded as a physical agent, atmospheric contagion has never been detected, and its presence has been inferred merely from the observation of what have been supposed its effects. It has certainly never been unequivocally manifested to any of the external senses. It has never been seen combined with the atmosphere, precipitated from it, or attracted therefrom, to solid bodies.

It might be supposed, however, from common parlance, that it has often made itself known to the sense of smell; but while nothing certainly proves that the impressions made on the nasal organ arise from atmospheric contagion, many circumstances induce at once the belief, that they proceed from common impurities.

The atmosphere in a sick chamber sometimes certainly has an odour, but it is certainly more logical to attribute this to the presence of impurities, whose presence there is no room to doubt, than to an agent whose existence under any circumstances has never been proven.

Had contagious matter the power of diffusing an odour through the air, it is probable, that would be constantly the same, in all cases of the same disease, and that each disease would have its own peculiar odour: but this correspondence is not found.

It is not desired to prove, that atmospheric contagion does not exist, because it cannot be detected by the senses.

Many agencies exist, which, under ordinary circumstances, are beyond the cognizance of the external senses; but in general they make themselves manifest to one, or other, under some conditions. The electricity of the air is neither seen nor felt under ordinary circumstances; but that agent is capable of being collected from the atmosphere in such quantities as are cognizable to the eye. Now, under any manner of circumstances, contagion has never been recognised by the senses—and it has never been detected by chemical experiments.

It is surely not unfair to expect, that, if a contagious poison, a palpable matter such as is contained in a small-pox pustule, is transformed to the vaporic state, or taken into the atmosphere, that the air so impregnated will be marked by some qualities, beyond those of simple, pure air. Perhaps air in which it is disseminated should have an odour, and perhaps that odour should be of a peculiar kind, in each disease. Should it not also be marked by some effects, constant and uniform, upon the human body, such as mark the career of such like agents in a palpable form, when applied either immediately, as by touch, or mediately, as by fomites? Perhaps it may not be deemed unreasonable to expect, that atmospheric contagion, did it exist, would produce its peculiar effects, as constantly, or nearly so, as a palpable contagious poison. But how different is the fact. If a hundred persons not formerly vaccinated, have the palpable contagion of cow-pox matter inserted under the skin, the probability is, that, if the matter is good, and the operation is skilfully done, 90 or 95 will be duly affected with the specific effects; whereas, when a hundred persons are exposed to the atmosphere of fever, and when these persons, too, have not before had the disease, perhaps not one, or at most not above two or three will take the distemper, unless the air has become extremely vitiated; and then the probability is, that it is so, not in consequence of the presence of specific contagious virus, but of gross impurities, and the consumption of the more vital parts, as in the case of the Black Hole of Calcutta, where putrid fever attacked all who survived their confinement, certainly not from the action of contagious poison.

CHAPTER V

Contagious Poisons—Non-Solution in the Air—Results of Experiments

Animal substances are the results of still more delicate processes, and of a more refined organization (than vegetables); and the balance of affinities, by which they exist, is disturbed by still slighter causes.

Henry

For the present, the argument drawn from the actual observation of the origin and propagation of disease, against the doctrine of atmospheric contagion, will be waived, and it is proposed here, before going farther, to inquire, whether the case may not be settled by a reference to the history of analogous agents, and to the results of experiment.

It is proposed here to inquire if it is likely, judging from their chemical constitution, that palpable contagious poisons, such as the matter of small-pox, may be disseminated through the air, without chemical changes being effected upon them, that must be destructive of their peculiar properties.

The palpable contagious poisons are products of the blood, formed therefrom, by the nicest processes. They partake of the nature common to all animal products; are, like them, prone to putrefaction,—and, like them, are of a very compound nature.

They are animal products: now it is a well known fact that almost all animal products are fixed—that is, incapable of being volatilized or disseminated in air, unchanged in chemical constitution.

Gelatin or animal jelly; albumen, or what is much the same, the white part of an egg; fibrin or muscular fibre, and the like, are never known to be in the vaporic state, or commingled with the air. They are incapable of assuming the aeriform state, not in virtue of a character peculiar to them, but on account of that nature they share in common with almost all animal principles, which precludes the possibility of their being volatilized. No experiment has ever been made which can show that the principles specified may be diffused through the air.

When exposed to the air for even a short period, decomposition takes place, and their original nature is totally subverted.

Their elements are held together by affinities too feeble to admit of their particles being separated by air, without new combinations being formed.

If heat be applied to them, immediate destruction takes place; if they be kept moist, and in merely a moderate temperature, putrefaction or fermentation, in the proper sense of the terms, occurs; if carefully dried and exposed to the atmosphere, they remain little altered, for a considerable time; but at length fundamental changes, though operating slowly, entirely change their nature.

It cannot be shewn that contagious poisons are less animalized than the products alluded to.

Is it ascertained that contagious poisons, unlike other proximate animal principles, enter into the aeriform state?

Putting aside the loose and rash statements current upon the subject, as unworthy of notice, there can be no doubt that, in the whole history of those poisons, no fact is known, that can legitimately be held as proving, that they possess such a property, or of giving the idea any degree of countenance.

On the other hand, many facts are known, which are adequate for the refutation of these statements, and that are sufficient to put the case beyond a doubt.

Small-pox propagates by a contagious poison, eliminated from the blood, and found in the pox or pustule.

It is known to every one that it affects, by contact, hence the practice of inoculation, which is nothing more than the inserting, under the skin, a little of that agent, a practice which has been in use among the negroes of Africa, since, or before, the introduction of the doctrines of Mahomet.

Many physicians, perhaps almost all, believe that it, the poison, may be diffused through the air, and in that situation produce its wonted effects; but evidence is submitted to shew, how questionable that is: and it is conclusive, as far as negative evidence can go.

The following experiment was performed by Dr O'Ryan of Lyons.[2] The force of its results, and their tendency, cannot be overlooked.

"A dish containing lint saturated with matter taken from the natural and the inoculated small-pox, was placed upon a table, whose diameter was three feet, and children who never had the disease, and never were inoculated or vaccinated, were placed around it, and kept there for some considerable time; yet none of them were seized with the disease."

"He also exposed children within two feet of a child affected at the time with the inoculated small-pox, for an hour daily, for fourteen days. None of the children were affected, and all were successfully inoculated two months afterwards."

We are acquainted, too, with many cases of small-pox, where the houses in which they were, were visited by many persons, some of whom had not been vaccinated, or inoculated, and yet the disease did not spread to them; and in those instances, where the distemper did spread, only some, and not all, who were liable, were affected, as would have been the case, had the matter been inserted under the skin.

Perhaps, in reference to this contagious matter and to others, it may be said that they were not favourably situated for acting. Heat, moisture, and the passing to and fro, of air, must certainly assist the assumption of the aeriform state; and a more favourable opportunity cannot be obtained, than the contagious matter of small-pox pustules has, in the mouth of the patient, where it almost always is observed. That situation is perhaps even more favourable than that of the matter operated on by Dr O'Ryan. Yet it is known, (and we are prepared to shew cases) that persons liable to the disease have breathed in the same apartment, and have not taken the distemper. We know, too, of many cases, where persons have been attacked under such circumstances, but that has probably arisen from actual contact with the matter, or exposure to those general and widely-spread influences productive of that pestilence, that undoubtedly exist. But it is

[2] O'Ryan, Sur les Fievres.

not necessary for our purpose, that all should escape, but, that any should not suffer. It is enough that those who escape, are more, in proportion, than those who resist the action of the palpable poison, when inserted into the system by inoculation.

With respect, also, to the disease produced by the insertion of cow-pox matter, or, in other words, by vaccination, as it is called; nobody ever heard of it being propagated through the air. It is feared that it would be a very inefficient mode of vaccinating, to bring the child to be vaccinated, into an atmosphere, to which was exposed an arm with a cow-pox. He who would propose such a plan would be laughed at by every old woman; and what is held as so absurd and ridiculous in respect to cow-pox, cannot be very wise in reference to small-pox, plague, scarlet fever, and the like. There are other diseases, too, which undoubtedly are propagated by palpable contagious poisons. Yet were any person affected with them, to whisper, that a contagious atmosphere had been the occasion, they would be held as using no small liberty with the credulity of the medical adviser.

There is yet another palpable contagious matter to which reference must be made,—that of itch. The only known way by which that disease can be propagated, from one to another, is by palpable or contactual contagion.

Many medical men are in the daily practice of seeing and examining such cases, yet they seldom or never are affected with it. Any caution directed against the operation of that contagion, is addressed exclusively to contact, never to the atmosphere.

The plague, according to the very best authorities, is undoubtedly marked by the elimination of a matter capable of producing the same pestilence, when applied in a palpable form, to the body of another. The plague has been produced intentionally by inoculation, and may be propagated at pleasure.

Dr Patrick Russell was satisfied, from the observation of much of that pestilence, that the atmospheric contagion did not extend the distance of four feet; and there is much room to think that, if he had extended his inquiry farther, that had he been aware how unusual it is for a proximate animal principle, as contagious matter, to take on the aeriform state, he would have arrived at the conclusion, that it did not only not exist, at the distance of four feet from the patient, but that it did not exist at all. Had he gone that length, he would not have created any more difficulties, to be explained away, than were made by laying down for it, such a limited range of operation, for there would, it seems, be little difficulty, in general, in discovering, that persons who had approached so near as four feet to the patient, had come in contact either with the sick himself, or the matter of the sores attached to clothes or other bodies.

We know of no facts capable of proving that the matter of plague is diffusible through the air; and the very evidence of Dr Russell, which was used by him to prove the limited range of atmospheric contagion, may be used to lend countenance to the position, that it does not exist at all.

The evidence was this:—Dr Russell was in the practice, at Aleppo, of examining plague sores from a window four feet from the patient, yet he suffered not from that pestilence.

Scarlet Fever is a disease universally held to be one of those propagated by a contagious principle.

It is commonly believed that a contagious poison is eliminated in the course of this disease, similar to that of small-pox.

Its history is marked by this remarkable feature, peculiar to acute contagious diseases, of attacking the same individual only once; and the disease is accompanied by a peculiar eruption, which may, without impropriety, be supposed to contain the said contagious poison. This eruption is uniform in the time of its appearance, its duration, and decay, like the other eruptions of other contagious diseases. On all these accounts, the Author is disposed to assent to its possession of the contagious poison;—and that will be taken for granted.

Connected with this view, is an observation made by Dr Sidey, of Edinburgh, in a paper contained in a late Number of the Edinburgh Medical and Surgical Journal, on Scarlatina, as lately prevalent in that town. It is to this effect, that he found that the disease, when characterized by a distinct eruption, attacked several members of a family more frequently, than when it wanted that symptom.

We will inquire whether persons exposed to an atmosphere containing one sick of that disease, take that distemper as uniformly, as those take the respective diseases of those palpable contagious poisons which may be inserted under the skin.

During a most severe and mortal visitation of that disease in Tranent and its surrounding country, which lasted from about the end of January to the 20th October 1836, many cases occurred, where brothers and sisters of children suffering under that malady, living in the same apartment, but not sleeping together, remained free of any attack whatever at the time.

Had the poison been capable of diffusion in the atmosphere, the air would have become highly contagious, and as persons were constantly inhaling it, and among them some liable to the disease, it would certainly have manifested its peculiar pestiferous influence upon them.

But the result was different, and the person exposed at that time remained quite free of it; and in the course of time, varying from weeks to several months after, went through the disease in the ordinary manner. These cases have been carefully noted and preserved.

But the Author was anxious to ascertain, by other means, whether that disease was capable of propagation by atmospheric contagion; and opportunities were not wanting.

It occurred that the matter of ulcers, in the throat, might possibly contain the contagious poison, and might be made the subject of experiment.

The following is a case in which the experiment was made.

The patient, a boy eight years old, had been exposed about three months before, constantly, to an atmosphere in which a younger brother, ill of scarlet fever, was breathing.

He had the precursory fever, and the tonsils and uvula (the parts at the back of the mouth) were almost covered with ash-coloured spots and suppurating ulcers.

A piece of linen, fixed to the extremity of a probe, was rubbed freely over the ulcers. The linen impregnated with matter and the secretions, was, within an hour or two of its being taken, exposed to the free action of the air of a small apartment, where it remained for ten days, without producing any effect, upon several persons, a good deal in the room; and among them, two children, one aged two, and the other fourteen years, who had not had scarlet fever. They respired the air occasionally and for a considerable time, on the several days.

The temperature was various. During the day being about 60° Fahr., and 40° during the night. The linen readily became dry, but was repeatedly moistened with water.

This experiment goes to shew, that the matter of the ulcers of scarlet fever is incapable of propagating the disease, through the medium of the air.

But scarcely any better nidus could be formed, for the dissemination of the matter, of the ulcers, through the atmosphere, than the sores themselves, the very place where it is eliminated; and cases have been referred to, where persons have respired an atmosphere thus liable to be acted on, with the most complete impunity.

It is not ascertained that the contagious poison is eliminated at the sores in the throat, but such seems probable, seeing that the sores are as essential and constant as the eruption itself.

Experiments might have been multiplied, but that has appeared unnecessary, as it is hoped that enough has been done to shew that the contagious poisons which have undergone our examination, are incapable of assuming the aeriform state, and, as it must seem probable, that in a point so important, they will all coincide, even those which have not been treated of here.

Their chemical constitution, as before remarked, prevents their assuming that state. Dr Henry of Manchester remarks, when pointing out the distinctive characters of animal and vegetable bodies, that "Animal substances are the results of still more delicate processes, and of a more refined organization, and the balance of affinities by which they exist is disturbed by still slighter causes;" and again says, "Instead of passing through the vinous and the acetous fermentation, they are peculiarly prone to undergo putrefaction."

Thus, then, this great law, ascertained and settled beyond

a doubt, and the results of our observations on the causes of diseases styled contagious, and of experiments on the palpable contagious poisons themselves, are opposed to the admission of this doctrine, and when we recall to memory the slender evidence, nay, the absence of any evidence at all, the conclusion almost necessarily is, that atmospheric contagion does not, and cannot exist.

With what justice may we now join with De Lolme, when he says—"There is a very essential consideration to be made in every science, though speculators are very apt to lose sight of it, which is, that in order that things may have existence, that they must be possible."

CHAPTER VII.

Contagious Poisons, Compared with Yeast—Does That Agent Assume the Aeriform State?

Lest the evidence we have laid before the reader should not be so satisfactory and conclusive as it has been deemed by us, the details and results of some investigation into yeast will now be given.

It occurred to us, that it would be useful, in our inquiry respecting contagious poisons, to ascertain whether or not yeast was capable of producing its wonted effects through the medium of the air, if, in short, it was capable of taking on the vaporic state. We were led to this inquiry from the consideration, that it and contagious poisons presented points of resemblance of the most important nature, and that the history of the one might elucidate that of the others.

Yeast is the only other inanimate substance, besides the contagious poisons, with which we are acquainted, which has the property of producing a substance in every respect like itself, in short, of reproduction.

Like the contagious poisons, too, it is the result of a great and active process, which, like them, it can again produce in other materials.

Fermentation may be likened to contagious disease, and, indeed, it is not the first time contagious disease has been likened to fermentation. These diseases produce contagious poisons,—fermentation produces yeast, and again, these agents produce their respective processes.

Bodies in general, which have undergone the action at least of the active contagious poisons, are not liable to be again affected by them; so vegetable bodies, which have undergone fermentation, by means of yeast, are not liable to be again acted upon by a second application.

It is important to know if yeast is capable of assuming the aeriform state.

It is a complex substance, being compound in its chemical constitution. Did we find that it was, then it might seem probable that contagious poisons (putting out of consideration the evidence already given), might possibly be so disseminated also. It runs readily into putrefaction, and in a short time loses its power of producing its peculiar effects, that is, fermentation.

Knowing this, we were inclined to believe that it could not get into the atmosphere otherwise than in a decomposed state, and, therefore, could not act through that medium.

The question was put to a most intelligent brewer, conversant with its common qualities, and the unhesitating answer was immediately given, that it could act through the air.

Here we could not help marking the striking similarity in the bearing of the brewer, with the confidence with which medical men speak of the like property of contagious poisons—the marked taking for granted *what* was opposed in both instances, to the obvious evidence of chemistry, and *what* might be so readily tested by experiment.

He was of opinion, that if fermentation were going on in a tub in an apartment where there was a quantity of wort (liquid ready for fermentation), to which no yeast had been added, that that process would be excited from the yeast in the fermenting tub, producing its influence through the medium of the atmosphere, in short, by being dissolved in it.

As that opinion did not tally with our opinions on chemical affinity, recourse was had to experiment.

1st Experiment.

A quantity of wort, to which no yeast had been added, was put into a wide mouthed vessel, and suspended in the mouth of a large tub, containing ale in an active state of fermentation. The vessel was allowed to remain three days, and at the end of that time no more appearance of fermentation was detected, than a very slight display of frothy bubbles in the middle, nothing more than we were assured by the brewer, was wont to appear from spontaneous fermentation.

A blind devotion to his opinion might have induced the

brewer to attribute to the yeast acting through the medium of the air, what was quite spontaneous, and if he had done so, how like his case would have been to that of some medical men, who unwittingly attribute to atmospheric contagion, what is spontaneous or dependent on other agencies.

From this experiment it appears that yeast is incapable of solution in the air, and of producing through that medium its peculiar effects.

But to make the result still more certain, another experiment was performed.

2d Experiment.

A wide mouthed vessel, containing a quantity of water, was suspended over some liquor, in a state of active fermentation, for the purpose of absorbing any gas or yeast, in a state of vapour proceeding from it. It was kept there two days, and then examined. Its taste was somewhat altered, and it had acquired a slight odour much resembling that of yeast, probably from the absorption of gas. It was thought, that if this water had become impregnated with yeast, that that circumstance would be rendered manifest, by producing fermentation, when added to a quantity of wort; and to determine the question, the following trial was made.

Two jugs half filled with wort, free from yeast, were placed in an apartment whose atmosphere was favourable to fermentation. To one was added the water which had been suspended over the fermenting tub, and to the other an equal quantity of pure water. They were then put aside, and secured from interference. At the end of three days they were examined. The wort to which had been added the water taken from over the fermenting tub, presented on its surface a few frothy bubbles, but not the slightest appearance of yeast.

The wort, to which pure water had been added, presented an appearance identically the same, having a few frothy bubbles on its surface, but not any other, the most trifling sign of fermentation.

Similar experiments were made at a distillery, where the facilities for their success were said to be even greater than at the brewery, and they were marked with precisely similar results.

Thus, then, it appears, as the result of experiment, that yeast is incapable of assuming the vaporic or aeriform state.

This inquiry will perhaps appear to many remote and unconnected with the proper subject of these pages, and, hence, that it is altogether superfluous; but we think differently, and are of opinion, that an accurate knowledge of that agent is calculated to be of the utmost use in forwarding the formation of a just estimate of the habitudes of the contagious poisons, which it resembles in several very important points.

It is, as before stated, the only other substance belonging to the inanimate world, whose immediate and most prominent property is that of propagating a substance identically the same—of producing, through a peculiar and uniform process, an agent possessed again of all its properties.

Some other agents may be said, under some circumstances, to propagate themselves, but it is in a very remote way, and by no means by that direct and uniform operation which marks the propagation of contagious poisons and yeast, which is obviously as well defined as germination among animal and vegetable bodies.

Heat, under some circumstances, does cause the production or evolution of heat, but that is rather an accidental circumstance, brought about remotely by the chemical operation produced, and would have taken place whatever had been the cause of that process, and is not the result of an immediate and particular property.

Vitiated air also is calculated much in the same way to reproduce itself; but, instead of being in virtue of a quality possessed by the palpable contagious poisons, vitiated air of itself produces disease, and a common result of disease is vitiated or impure air.

The close analogy subsisting between yeast and the palpable contagious poisons, it is hoped, has been fully made out; and though it is not permitted, by the rules of logic, positively to determine, that the laws which regulate the action of the one, necessarily hold with the other agents; yet, where there is no evidence of a contrary nature, the closeness of the connection lends countenance to the idea.

That analogy seems remarkably strong when it is considered, that both yeast and the palpable contagious poisons produce their peculiar effects only once upon the same object.

Many instances are known where the palpable contagious poisons have produced their peculiar effects more than once, but these deserve rather to be held as exceptions to the general law than as a proof against its existence.

Part II

Chapter I

The Negation of Atmospheric Contagion from the History and Actual Observation of Disease

Ce qu'il y'a d'extraordinaire c'est que ceux qui fatiguent leur raison pour lui faire rapporter de certains événements à des vertus occultes n'ont pas un moindre effort à faire pour s'empêcher d'en voir la véritable cause.

Montesquieu.

It has been attempted, in the preceding part of this work, to prove, on general principles, and by a reference to analogous objects, that atmospheric contagion cannot exist; but, lest that object should appear unaccomplished, and that the data are insufficient for the conclusion proposed, it is purposed to test the merits of the question by the consideration of the history and phenomena of disease.

Those circumstances, connected with the appearance and propagation of disease, on which the doctrine of atmospheric contagion rests, will be inquired into, and their weight and importance duly ascertained. This inquiry will be prosecuted as if no such investigation as the preceding had been made, and as if the existence of that agency was not irreconcilable with well ascertained laws; and, for the sake of argument, the possibility of its existence will be conceded.

The facts in the history of disease, which are held as lending countenance to the doctrine of atmospheric contagion—of proving its existence, are, chiefly, the general prevalence of disease at one and the same time among the members of the same family, of the inhabitants of the same town, district, and country,—its affecting the visitors and attendants of the sick,—and its observation in places hitherto healthy, shortly after communication with those ravaged with the distemper. These facts cannot be denied; and all that can be done is to weigh their value, as proofs of the existence of atmospheric contagion, and the first mentioned will occupy our attention.

THE EVIDENCE DRAWN FROM THE WIDELY SPREAD AND SIMULTANEOUS PREVALENCE OF DISEASE, IN FAVOUR OF ATMOSPHERIC CONTAGION, CONSIDERED.

The widely-spread prevalence of disease at the same time among the inhabitants of a country or district, is almost invariably held as affording proof of the presence and operation of atmospheric contagion.

The ravages of pestilence, rapid, wide, and deadly, are noticed in the histories of all nations, and at intervals they have been experienced during the long period of the existence of the world; and the destruction of whole armies, and the annihilation of entire nations, prove how widely spread its operation has sometimes been.

Did the circumstance of disease being widely spread prove its propagation by atmospheric contagion, then the matter were at rest; but the propriety of such an inference is questionable.

Let it be supposed that there is prevailing, in a district of country, disease to a great amount, that is to say, many cases of the same distemper.

That single circumstance proves nothing in reference to atmospheric contagion, more than to any other probable cause of disease. It shews, merely, that there is in wide operation some cause or causes of sickness; and it is totally unwarrantable to conclude that one agency, more than another, is the efficient cause, without further information directly bearing on the subject.

It is with the knowledge of the single fact, and in total ignorance of others, or with total blindness to them, that atmospheric contagion is pronounced to be the active agent.

Now it is not the peculiar property, the exclusive prerogative of that principle, to cause disease; at least, that character has not been openly sought by its advocates, though the tone of common conversation, and of medical writings on the subject, would seem to imply that it had been tacitly granted.

That cannot be conceded. Many other agencies are known to be productive of sickness, and have, on many occasions, induced pestilence of a deadly character, that has ravaged in no despicable limits.

The isolated fact itself of disease being widely extended in the absence of particulars, after proving that some cause existed, should legitimately go to create a suspicion, that the cause or causes which had produced the first cases, and acted as the ordinary springs of the malady, were continuing to operate on other individuals. Such would be known to be capable of producing the effect observed, for the satisfactory reason, that it or they had already accomplished it. How much more wise, under such circumstances, it would be to suspect the continuance of that influence with the continuance of effects identically the same as it or they had already produced, than to call in a principle whose only evidence of existence was the presence of effects, the same as had been only a short time before produced by a different agency, and of whose removal or absence there was not a particle of proof.

But a little inquiry will, on most occasions, elicit the fact, that some pestiferous influences exist; and it will, in general, be soon enough to pronounce on the probable causes of a distemper after that investigation has been made.

Disease in general, unconnected with alterations in the texture of the organs, is neither more nor less than a derangement of the functions performed by the body; and as it partakes of a general or local character, so the disease is either local or general; and, as it relates to functions, more or less important, so it is more or less dangerous.

It must be obvious, that a machine so nicely balanced, so complicated and so exquisitely wrought as the human body, must be liable, on many occasions, to have its operations impeded and deranged; and, although sometimes said to be a little world of itself, still, it is dependent on surrounding agencies. It requires a pure atmosphere for respiration, food to supply the waste it continually suffers, and drink to appease thirst, and to take the place of the fluids that are constantly draining from it.

The human body is necessarily brought in contact with

the external world; and many are the injuries it suffers therefrom, both directly and remotely.

The derangements of the functions of the body are in general owing to circumstances of an unwholesome character, for the most part relating to food, drink, the various steps in nutrition, the atmosphere, its temperature, dryness, moistness, purity, &c. &c., and chemical and mechanical agents, to whose action the body is exposed.

Were it not for the operation of unfavourable circumstances of the nature specified, a body in health, were no special interposition of the Almighty hand made, would go on in the healthy performance of its functions, till the frailty and decay, incident to old age, would overtake it.

In general those diseases which are observed to prevail to a great extent, and over a large tract of country at the same time, are so uniformly coincident with circumstances of an unwholesome tendency, connected with those agencies above referred to, that they appear at once to the candid and unprejudiced inquirer, to stand in the relation of cause and effect. Surely it should cause no difficulty, nor occasion any necessity for the calling in a principle, atmospheric contagion, without any other evidence, that those effects are occasionally found not confined to one spot merely, but are seen developed in an extended sphere—for, assuredly, it can require no extraordinary effort of the mind to conceive that the agent acting and causing disease in one place, or individual case, may with equal force, and with a like result, act in many situations, and in respect to many persons.

The presence of certain operations in several situations by no means proves that they have reproduced themselves.

Day-light is manifest in many countries, within certain latitudes at the same hour, but it has never been suggested that this circumstance in one of them has been propagated by that of another, through any occult principle, or whatever else such an agency may be called.

Had the case not presented at once, and in so direct and striking a manner, a sufficient cause for the effects observed, then we doubt not, that, perhaps, individuals would relieve themselves of any present difficulty, and attribute what they could not readily explain, to the operation of a principle having as little evidence of its entity as atmospheric contagion itself. But the sun is too glorious, too resplendent an object to be overlooked, and its effects are too immediate, to permit the possibility of the most unreflecting, not marking its relation as cause to the effect observed.

But, unfortunately, the relation between widely spread diseases or epidemics, as they are called, and circumstances connected with the agencies before referred to, is not so striking—though it is as close. There is no object so bright to draw the same attention to it, and to proclaim it from east to west, from the dawn of morning till the fall of evening, like that luminary dispersing light as he appears to traverse the heavens.

Yet there is room to believe that the presence of epidemics is always accompanied, or shortly preceded, by circumstances, which, though by reason of their less striking character, and less immediate operation, are sometimes overlooked or neglected, yet do exist, and, were inquiry made by those able for the purpose, doubtless would be found.

In most of the epidemics recorded, some such agencies or circumstances were in operation. They were known to be so—and in almost all that have come under our own observation, and they have neither been few nor carelessly noted—there have, on nearly every occasion, been found the influences to which we allude.

We are led to believe an agent to be the cause of an effect when the one follows upon the operation or presence of the other, uniformly, and on every occasion, when the latter bears some relation in its amount to the force and length of duration of the former—and when the effect ceases with the removal of the agent. Such a close connection, as subsists in that case, entitles the former or agent to be held as the cause of the effect observed.

For those very reasons day-light is said to be the effect of the sun that comes with it, remains with it, and goes with it.

Let us see if the same connection holds with disease and those agencies and circumstances we have cursorily referred to.

Those agencies and circumstances, relating to food,

drink, air, heat, contagious matter, &c. &c. are known to present themselves, and with them are presented diseases. They are known to remain, and with them are known to continue diseases. They are known to disappear, and with them all the world knows diseases disappear also.

These being the causes of epidemic or widely spread disease, as such a connection proves, it is altogether superfluous to admit the operation of atmospheric contagion, whose existence has never been known, but by the very circumstances which it is said to bring about.

It is surely most unwise, when we see disease arising with the existence of unwholesome circumstances, such as scarcity of food, unwholesome quality of it, great vicissitudes of weather, uncommon conditions of the atmosphere, want of sufficient clothing or incommensurate with the severities of the season, the operation of depressing passions, and the like,—growing with their intensity—extending where they extend—abating where they decrease—and finally disappearing when they disappear—to refuse to grant the relation as cause and effect, and to plunge into the tide of difficulties such ill-timed incredulity creates, with nothing but the appearance, nothing but the assurance, of an object to grasp at.

In general, such a connection can be made out between the existence of wide-spread disease and such circumstances.

If, in respect to some diseases, so intimate a connection cannot be observed, the probability is, that it is the obscurity connected with these subjects, the less direct way in which they operate and the remote time at which their effects may be experienced on the body, that are the occasion of the difficulty. The human body, unlike mere inanimate matter, has the power of withstanding, at least for a time, the operation of unwholesome influences, if not very virulent; and it is only natural to allow, that, in respect to a machine so complicated, affected by so many agencies, and standing in so many relations, there will be less complete directness of operation, than with simple or inanimate substances, and more variety in the amount and duration of the effect.

On these accounts, the indications of the case are less direct and obvious, and it should cause no great surprise, that being considered, and the fact of the imperfect state of our knowledge on the varieties of the agencies referred to, being kept in mind, that the causes of disease cannot at all times be completely and satisfactorily ascertained.

Our knowledge of the derangements of health, from the operation of these agencies, on some of which we are dependent, and with others of which we are constantly brought in contact, is fast increasing, and the relation between the former and the varieties in the latter is becoming clear and precise. There is, therefore, reason to hope that difficulties which now baffle us, will soon be explained away, and that much of that mist that has long overhung the causes of pestilence, will soon be dissipated.

Certain circumstances produce certain uniform effects, and in every instance where they are operating, their effects will be produced, provided no agency is acting adequate to neutralize them. Not one hill only, in northern latitudes, has its summit whitened with snow, nor does sterility mark a few spots only in the immense deserts of Africa and Asia.

The same features are spread far and wide. They owe their existence to agencies acting in immense spheres corresponding with their own.

The sphere of those circumstances connected with the agents so often referred to, that produce disease, is sometimes large, and no astonishment need be felt, if that of disease is also large, since a relation ever holds between the extent of a cause and its effects.

It would certainly be ample time to call in the assistance of atmospheric contagion to account for the propagation of disease, when its sphere or circle is found to be positively eccentric of that of those circumstances alluded to.

But we are satisfied that such a contingency is of very rare occurrence, and even when it is said to exist, we shall require some undoubted assurance that the non-correspondence is not the result of ignorance of the extent of these hurtful circumstances, rather than the actual absence of relation between them.

It is not our intention at present to enlarge on the causes of disease, yet we maintain, that such a relation as that referred to, will in almost every instance be made out, if candid and efficient inquiry be instituted; so that, even granting that atmospheric contagion exists, there can be no room for its operation. And we are of opinion, that if, in some extraordinary instance, no such relation can be detected, the progress which every department of science is making will in time achieve what may not be accomplished at present.

The history of nations and the records of medicine shew, that, coincident with epidemic sickness, there have, for the most part, been noticed certain circumstances operating which were prejudicial to the welfare of the human body. For example, famine, bad or unwholesome food, great and long continued droughts, great rains followed by intense heat, sudden vicissitudes of weather, dissipation, irregularities, depressed state of mind, insufficient clothing and fuel, and unwholesome water.

These, and many similar circumstances known to prevail in the haunts of pestilence, must exert a great, a very powerful, influence on the human body, and, when the question of the probable causes of its diseases is mooted, it argues a strange and discreditable blindness to obvious facts, to overlook the part which they must exert in their production; and a strong and dangerous partiality to a questionable principle, to attribute the whole calamity to atmospheric contagion.

CHAPTER II

The Evidence Drawn from Disease Attacking the Relatives, Attendants, and Visitors of the Sick, in Favour of Atmospheric Contagion, Considered—Facts Explained

Few points have been held so conclusive of the existence of atmospheric contagion, as the circumstance of the attendants and visitors of the sick being attacked with the same distemper, during, or shortly after, their communication.

It is vain to deny, that where a person is ill of a disease, such as fever, that those about him, the members of his family, his attendants, and his visitors, are sometimes attacked with the same distemper.

Such is a common occurrence, but common as it is, it cannot prove that the efficient cause is atmospheric contagion.

Were it established that atmospheric contagion existed in that individual disease, and in that individual case, then it might be admitted that the circumstance did lend some countenance to the supposition, and should perhaps entitle the case to examination.

But it has never been shown that that principle positively exists. There is, as has already been observed, no proof, saving that drawn from the very circumstances for which it is called in to account.

Thus it is entitled to no exclusive respect.

Here is then an agency, of whose existence there is no evidence of a sufficient nature, and here there is reason to believe that the same circumstances are operating widely, and upon the relatives, the attendants, and visitors of the sick, which have already produced the disease in those visited.

These circumstances, in general, are ascertained to be acting upon these individuals, and where they cannot, from their obscure nature, be recognised, there is reason, from the very circumstance of the sick having been affected, to conclude that they are operating, though perhaps in an insidious way. Now, a question arises, whether it is wisest to attribute the prevalence of disease among those holding communication with the sick, to the operation of atmospheric contagion, or to those circumstances and agencies which caused the disease originally, and which there is room to believe are exerting their influence over them also.

It has been said in the preceding chapter, that, during the prevalence of widely spread or epidemic disease, there are generally found circumstances of an unwholesome tendency, favouring its career, and that the range of their action corresponds with that of pestilence. That being the case, as it undoubtedly is, it would be proper, before admitting the operation of atmospheric contagion, to shew that no such circumstances were in operation. An inquiry would be necessary; and their presence being proven, it would not be short of imbecility to attribute to that agency, effects such as are wont to follow their action. It would be to call in a principle whose existence has never been proven, and which, therefore, must be held as at least doubtful, to account for phenomena, the ordinary results of circumstances present, which would indeed be absurd.

Before the operation of atmospheric contagion could with propriety be entertained, it behoved to shew that those circumstances which induced disease in the visited, were not operating with those holding communication with them.

But in all those cases in which atmospheric contagion is held as acting, no attempt is made to prove such absence, and the belief in its presence is not the less strong because these circumstances can be proved to be present.

It is a self-evident truth that some agency or agencies, totally independent of atmospheric contagion must have been in operation, and acting as the cause of disease in the first case or cases that occurred. For this ample reason, that, for atmospheric contagion to exist at all, it is obviously necessary that disease pre-existed, since it is the product of disease, and of disease only.

Thus, then, it is proved, that some causes, totally independent of atmospheric contagion, produce the first cases of an epidemic, or widely spread disease. Now, there is no evidence that these same causes are not operating upon those who visit the sick, and in absence of any facts to the contrary, and of the operation of an equally active and undoubted agent, there is justice in thinking it probable that they are acting, more especially if the self-same results are manifested—and this may, with safety, be done, even when direct testimony cannot be obtained—which is very seldom entirely the case.

The causes of the disease being widely extended, and the visited patient being ill from the operation of forces shared in common with many, it is only fair to conclude that as relatives, attendants, and visitors are like the great mass of people thus operated upon—that they, *cæteris paribus*, are as likely to be affected with the prevalent disease, as those who are suffering were previous to its invasion.

They do suffer, but not in general in a greater proportion than other persons having no communication, and similarly situated in other respects.

It would be ample time to look for the operation of some other agency in addition to those commonly experienced, when the portion of the community, holding communication with the sick, is affected with disease in a greater proportion than that portion having none.

Now, with a few exceptions, it is the result of much patient investigation, not only into the experience of others, but of many epidemics we have had the most ample means of noting, that, in general, in respect to diseases held to be propagated by atmospheric contagion, those who have communication with the sick, do not suffer in a greater proportion than those who keep apart, but remain in the sphere in which the agencies and circumstances are operating, which produced the first cases.

These exceptions are—

1st, The relations and inmates of the same house inhabited by one sick of fever.

2d, Those receiving disease from actual contact with the palpable contagious matter, or by contactual contagion.

3d, Those persons, through the operation of fear, and from depression of mind, affected with disease, as fever, cholera, &c.

4th, The attendants in fever institutions, &c.

These exceptions will meet with a little consideration, in order to shew in what manner, and wherefore, those persons are seized in greater proportion, and to prove that it is not in consequence of atmospheric contagion.

This statement is important, and is made cautiously, and only after the most detailed examination, and unprejudiced weighing of evidence.

The facts which have led to that conclusion might be detailed, but, as they would occupy much room, and perhaps prove uninteresting to the general reader, they will be withheld, however, to be produced, if any sufficient objections be made.

That statement is contrary to common belief, which attributes disease in a much greater proportion to those communicating with the sick, than to those keeping apart; but that is not of much consequence, since implicit reliance is not to be placed upon the opinions on that subject, held either by the public or the medical profession.

On the whole, disease does affect, in a greater ratio, those who communicate with the sick, than those who do not, the instances which we excepted being included. But the difference, on the whole, is very trifling, at least much less than is usually supposed.

One of the reasons that the difference is thought to be much more than is actually the case, is, that every case of a visitor or attendant being affected with disease, after or during communication, is bruited about, and becomes the subject of much gossip; while that of hundreds, equally exposed, who escape, is treated very judiciously with silence. There is no impartial hearing of evidence. All that is heard is taken in favour of one side, and instead of an opinion being formed from the whole bearings of the case, one is got up on partial statements, which, however, as it agrees with preconceived notions, answers very well.

But that is not the way in which a case so important should be treated. Be it hoped that medical men, at least, will take more enlarged views, when their own reputation and the public weal are at stake.

The partial statements remind us strongly of the self-deception of which many persons are the dupes, in respect to fortune-telling and the solving of dreams. Every instance of the divination of the fortune-teller, or the solution of a dream, having any, the most far-fetched, correspondence with the future history of the individual, is stored up in the memory, and adduced as undeniable evidence of the truth of those dark arts, however much a thousand facts may cry out against them as vile impositions. The prognostications must, of necessity, be right sometimes, in much the same manner as Louis the 14th declared those astrologers must at some time be correct, who were constantly foretelling his death.

We now proceed to inquire into the circumstances which cause disease to attack those having communication with the sick, in a greater proportion than is observed to hold with those apart from them, yet living in the sphere of the epidemic causes, that is, generally speaking, in the same locality.

Exception 1st, The greater proportion in which relatives and others inhabiting the same house with one sick of disease, are attacked, we would explain in this manner:—

1st, The relatives, if inhabiting the same locality, are, like others, liable to the disease.

They are suffering in general under depression from apprehension of losing a dear friend.

They are, perhaps, under an apprehension that they themselves may be affected with the same distemper. They may have a dread of atmospheric contagion, or, as is often the case, may have a presentiment of fatal sickness.

They are irregular in the time of taking diet—have often no appetite—are deprived of their night's rest—maintain long and anxious watchings—and are in general in that feverish state of mind that precludes the possibility of taking due rest.

They are deprived of their wonted exercise in the open air, and of that elasticity of mind and body which it imparts.

They respire an atmosphere, though not contagious, often, and especially in the houses of the poor, deprived of its oxygen or more important principle, and tainted with the admixture of adventitious vapours or gases arising from the excretions, and perhaps the fermenting of impurities often found collected on the skin.

It would be wonderful, where there is a widely-spread disposition to disease, say to fever, if members of the same family, inhabiting the same house, in which one of them lay ill of that distemper, did not take ill, seeing how much they are exposed to it.

Nor is it to be thought extraordinary that relatives living in the same locality, but in different houses, or even in different villages, should take the disease also after visiting the house of a sick friend. What has been stated will sufficiently explain that occurrence.

Here it will perhaps be permitted to make a slight digression to mention a fact which has given much credit to the doctrine of atmospheric contagion,—the simultaneous invasion of fever among relatives, living together, in different houses, in different villages, and in very different parts of the country. We are aware of several extraordinary instances, where from ten to twenty of the same family were ill, at the same time, of fever, several of whom were living far apart.

It is in vain to think of atmospheric contagion being the cause. Possibly that notion might be entertained in reference to those living together, and having communication,—but cannot possibly apply to those in remote and different parts of the country. We know of instances where a family has been seized with fever in our village, and members of the same, living at great distances, forty and sixty miles, have suffered the same distemper at or nearly at the same time, without any communication having subsisted, either by person, by packets, or by letter.

These extraordinary circumstances speak of something more than atmospheric contagion. That could not possibly have extended to those relatives who had no communication; and it is remarkable that, in those instances, disease did not go as with the other members of the community, attacking at leisure, now this, now that one, but almost on the same day, many different members of the same family.

We have sometimes thought, from the consideration of such circumstances, that there is something like a community of disposition causing members of the same family to be similarly affected by like agents, more than subsists between men who are unconnected:—something like an idiosyncrasy, which goes to make them suffer after the same fashion.

There are such things as family characters, family idiosyncracies, family dispositions, family peculiarities of bodily conformation, and family temperaments; and may there not exist some family disposition, to be similarly affected by like circumstances?

The case appears well worthy of philosophical inquiry, something beyond the untenable puerilities of Mesmerians.

2d Exception.—Visitors and attendants are liable to increase their ordinary chance of taking the prevalent distemper, by touching the body or clothes of the sick, when he labours under a disease marked by a palpable contagious poison. Though the poison cannot be diffused through the air, it may, and sometimes does, act by contact, which we call contactual or immediate contagion. That, of course, can operate in those diseases only in which a palpable poison is eliminated. Those diseases are in this country chiefly small-pox, chicken-pox; the plague, if it can now be said to be a disease of this country; the itch; and, as is commonly believed, measles, scarlet fever, &c. &c.

Though the propagation of these diseases may take place from contact with their peculiar contagious matters, we are disposed to think, that, at least with most of them, especially the latter, the cases which occur in that way are very few.

It is sometimes difficult to produce disease, even when the skin is cut, and the matter is then introduced. That step sometimes fails in respect to cow-pox matter, even when fresh; and small-pox matter we have known to be in contact with the tips of the finger for a minute or so, in innumerable cases, as in feeling the pulse, and no disease has followed. Women affected with small-pox bear healthy children.

Almost the only diseases which we are disposed to think are propagated by contact with the person or clothes of the sick, are small-pox, chicken-pox, scabies, plague, &c. They all possess palpable matters in abundance.

Many instances are known to us, where children have got small-pox, and of grown-up people who have got itch, from sleeping with those sick of these distempers, and thus coming in contact with them closely, and for some time; and where they have not been seized with them, when only breathing the same atmosphere used by those sick.

Thus visitors and attendants may get disease by contact with palpable contagious matter, that is, by contactual contagion, and by touching clothes impregnated with the same, that is, by fomitic contagion, which they would not have taken, had they merely been respiring the air used by the patients.

3d Exception.—The visitors, and those in general holding communication with the sick, are also liable to be affected more with disease than others who remain free of it, on account of the sorrow usually felt on all occasions of public calamities, and particularly of very mortal pestilence, and more especially experienced in all its acuteness, in the silent sick-room of a friend.

Among the scenes our professional duties call us to witness, there is, perhaps, none so touching as the sorrow-striken countenances of friends, directed to the sick, nay, perhaps the deathbed of one they love; and we have noted the unspeakable sorrow then felt, the deep anguish then experienced, and the silence more touching than eloquence that reigns throughout the sick-room, as an awful contemplation, truly indicative of a depression that is calculated to throw its sufferers into the same situation which they so much deplore in others.

That sorrow attendant on such calamities, and that was so well marked, when cholera lately assailed the nations of the earth, throws into the shade almost every other form, sinks deep into the soul, and enervates every principle of life. It gives a pall to every taste, a disregard to all enjoyment, deprives the unhappy victim of that serenity and composure so favourable to health, and, on the contrary, imparts a restlessness to body and mind, until at length his system becomes a very nidus of disease.

None who have attentively watched the course of widely-spread disease, can doubt that that sorrow, so generally experienced on those occasions, is an active instrument, and a strong abettor of the original epidemic influences. It must be obvious to them, that those strong and deeply-felt emotions, with which man contemplates his relatives, his neighbours, aye, his very race, falling around him,—feeling, too, that he is in the midst of danger, and can do nothing for his security,—must produce a withering influence on the most vital functions of the body, and prove the immediate cause of disease.

Under such circumstances, when disease manifests itself, it certainly cannot be wise to disregard the part they must enact in the production of the effect observed, and to attribute the whole, or nearly the whole, to the operation of atmospheric contagion, which has already been shewn to be without sufficient evidence of its existence, in any one case, or in any one disease.

The visitors, also, are exposed to the action of an atmosphere, which, as it is sometimes impure, is liable to be hurtful.

4th Exception.—That of the attendants in Fever Institutions. It has often been remarked, that in some fever institutions the nurses and medical clerks resident in the house, are attacked with fever in a much greater ratio than holds with the population around. The difference has been seen on some occasions to be very great, and from information collected on the subject, we are disposed to think, on some occasions, and in reference to some institutions at least, that the statement is correct. That fact has been attributed to atmospheric contagion; and we shall proceed to inquire if it is not more likely that it is dependent on other circumstances which are operating, and that are known to be adequate for the effect observed.

The history of the Royal Infirmary of Edinburgh, and of Queensberry House, an institution for the reception of fever patients, shews that on some occasions almost all the clerks and nurses waiting upon those affected with fever, have been seized with it also.

And it would appear to be owing to some agency peculiar to fever patients or their wards; for in regard to the first-mentioned institution, it is ascertained that it is with those attendants only, who wait upon those patients, that the greater amount of sickness is experienced. Those attendants exclusively occupied in the surgical wards being attacked in no greater proportion than those unconnected with the institution.

This is certainly an important fact, and one on which the advocates of atmospheric contagion are wont to place no small weight. Did that principle exist, there is perhaps no fact in the whole history of medicine, on which we would place more reliance in proving its operation, for it is self-evident that nothing relating to the general unwholesomeness of the institution can be entitled to much activity in this case, for any insalubrious tendency of its situation, of the soil on which it stands, or emanations therefrom, and of the general economy and discipline, cannot be confined in their operation to one apartment or ward, cannot possibly be experienced in the fever wards only.

But an occurrence of this kind is apt to be too readily received and made the ground of many inferences. In itself it certainly is a strong, a cogent fact, and such as naturally leads the mind to believe, that, as some very potent agency is at work, it may be that of atmospheric contagion, which in alleged activity is surpassed by none.

Before proceeding to explain the occurrence, on principles very different from atmospheric contagion, it is right to say that it is such as does not occur in connection with all such institutions; and that, if the case which has been stated, proves it is likely such a principle as contagion is present in these institutions, that others of a directly opposite nature, and as much to the purpose, can be produced to shew, granting the possibility, that it is not present in other institutions, much larger.

By physicians of the first eminence, such occurrences as that referred to in connection with the Royal Infirmary of Edinburgh, are held as decisive proof of the operation of contagious atmosphere.

Dr Alexander Tweedie, a physician of London, and one justly eminent, after mentioning the self-same cause, goes on to say, in a sufficiently assured tone,—"No statement more conclusive, as to the contagious nature of fever, need be adduced: and if such facts will not lead to conviction, the mind of such a sceptic must be strangely constructed indeed."

The case had been made much stronger, and would have stood inquiry much better, had Dr Tweedie shewn, that the occurrence he treats of was not solitary or uncommon, but was such as is wont to be observed in all like institutions.

He should have known, that it is not from extraordinary, nor even from unique cases alone, that knowledge is to be obtained, nor laws deduced, of the ordinary characters, and action of disease. It is dangerous to deduce inferences, and construct laws, from the knowledge of one circumstance, and where, too, many can be obtained bearing on the case.

Let us see if this occurrence holds with other establishments. We will find that it by no means always holds.

Dr Bateman, who saw much of fever, and gave it much of his active consideration, in his excellent Treatise on Contagious Fever, says,—"During the fourteen years, in the course of which I have almost daily been in contact with persons labouring under contagious fever, not only myself, but all the nurses have been preserved from infection, with one exception, down to the period of the present epidemic" (in the London House of Recovery).[3]

Similar cases of exemption might be given, but it seems unnecessary to say more here.

But though Dr Bateman's evidence in a manner meets the case recorded, connected with the Royal Infirmary of Edinburgh, yet it does not disprove its correctness; and we proceed to explain what has been held as only to be explained by the presence of atmospheric contagion.

But though the case could not at present be explained, we deny that one such circumstantial piece of evidence should outweigh the many facts, and the results of reasoning, that have been laid before the reader, and that are yet to follow.

When evidence is contradictory, it is well to ascertain on which side it preponderates; and even when it is nicely balanced, which is not the case here, it should be tested by a reference to general principles. That was done in the first part

[3] Bateman on Contagious Fever, p. 154. 1818.

of this work, and the reader cannot have forgotten the result.

We are disposed to think, that the great prevalence of fever among the nurses and resident medical attendants of fever institutions, and fever wards in general hospitals, which does occasionally occur, is, in no small degree, owing to the particularly great contamination of the atmosphere, which is liable to take place from the peculiarly strong tendency there is in the body of those labouring under fever, especially of the low or typhoid character, to run to putrescence.

The body, it is ascertained, so afflicted, is particularly prone to putrefaction, as is sufficiently attested by the presence of black spots upon the surface, sordes upon the teeth and gums, and the general appearance of corruption, often sufficiently manifest.

The secretions and excretions are marked at first by a putrid character, and in a short time they are in an active state of putrefaction. In that state, chemical changes take place, gases are evolved, such as nitrogen, hydrogen, carbureted hydrogen, phosphureted hydrogen, singly and combined, forming for instance ammonia, which is a combination of hydrogen and nitrogen: they become mingled with the atmosphere, and impart to it pestiferous qualities.

In fever, the body is much more prone to run into the state of putrefaction, than when in health, or even when affected with merely local disease. The whole system is then affected, the whole functions are deranged, the decayed parts of the blood and solids are not removed, nor are they corrected by admixture with new and purer elements obtained from the products of digestion. The correcting influence of exercise is lost, and likewise the assistance it gives to the due performance of the various secretions; and it need not cause surprise that a body so situated, for days and weeks, becomes at length prone to putrefaction.

It will perhaps be argued, that the same corruption or contamination of the air is as likely to take place in the surgical wards, where patients are kept having sores, &c. But in those wards, in general, there is not the same amount of tendency to putrefaction. Their health is often excellent, their functions are often not at all deranged, and their bodies, in general, are not more prone to putrefaction than those in health.

There are, to be sure, a multitude of sores and the like, but, as long as they are healthy, and the matter is good, there is no risk of their injuring the air, provided they are kept tolerably clean.

Healthy matter is a bland and innocent fluid, not more prone to putrefaction than healthy blood. When healthy, matter may be present in an apartment or ward in abundance, without the least injury being felt by those respiring the atmosphere in the room in which it is contained, as the history of surgical hospitals amply proves.

But as soon as matter, by any means, becomes of a bad character, acrid, fretting, unkind, and prone to putrefaction, then it sends forth gases, and perhaps, compound agents, produced by their combination, which mingle with the atmosphere, impart to it most virulent properties, and thus produce havoc among the various patients, as great, as well marked, and as dreadful as those sometimes observed among the attendants of fever patients, from the supposed operation of what has been considered atmospheric contagion.

Wounds are much connected with the state of the general health. Where that, by any means, is affected in a serious manner, the wound takes on an unhealthy aspect, and the matter, which before was bland, becomes acrid and irritating. If the body is affected with a putrid taint, then the matter takes on the same, and from the emanations spoken of, disease spreads around the ward.

That dreadful disease, called hospital gangrene, was some years ago a common affection in military hospitals, from effluvia, and inattention to ventilation; and it was common to observe healthy wounds taking on a sphacelating character, from such causes. Sir John Pringle says, "I have seen instances of it (hospital fever), beginning in a ward, where there was no other cause, but one of the men having a mortified leg."[4]

There are other circumstances of a hurtful character, operating in general upon the young gentlemen who fill the offices of clerks, and upon the nurses, in these

[4] Sir John Pringle on Diseases of the Army, p. 288.

establishments, which we doubt not co-operate with the other circumstances mentioned, in producing the extraordinary amount of disease sometimes observed among them. But of these which will readily suggest themselves to all, it is unnecessary to say much in this place.

It is in the fever wards principally that contagious atmosphere is apprehended.

The young gentlemen officiating as clerks are generally arrived at the most important part of their course of study. They are in preparation for their examination before the colleges, and are often in consequence in a very feeble state of health—which, if not always marked with actual sickness, is often sufficiently indicated by worn out and emaciated systems, and by complexions of a very sallow or sickly colour. They are thus predisposed to fever. The nurses waiting upon fever patients are subject to more fatigue and more interruptions to their rest, on account of the great attention which those under their care require, than the same class of persons are exposed to, who belong to the surgical wards.

Chapter III

The Argument Drawn in Favour of the Propagation of Disease by Atmospheric Contagion, from Disease Appearing in Previously Healthy Houses and Localities to which Persons Sick, or Lately So, Have Been Removed

A case of an apparently strong nature is made out in favour of the propagation of disease by atmospheric contagion, when a person labouring under sickness or lately recovered from it, is removed into a house or locality in which the same malady shortly manifests itself. It is often held conclusive; we hold it otherwise.

Such a case is known to take place, and we have observed it in our own practice—but that is not entitled to be considered conclusive. It should be shewn, if that inference is at all to be arrived at, that the occurrence is so frequent that the probability is precluded of attributing the phenomena observed to the ordinary causes of disease, that the number who thus suffer is greatly more in proportion than holds among the population generally, and that, in short, those thus visited by the sick are affected in a greater ratio than holds with the general community, as ascertained by an observation of the whole course of the disease or epidemic.

We know that the appearance of disease among those visited by the sick, or those lately recovered, does not always happen. We ourselves, scarcely recovered of typhus fever, have visited and lived with a family at a distance, and no such thing as propagation has occurred—and hundreds of other cases are within our knowledge. We have, after making calculations on the subject, considering both those cases, where disease did occur and where it did not, that, generally speaking, those visited by convalescents, or even patients, suffer in a proportion very little greater, if at all greater, than those having no such intercourse—compared of course with the very many cases that are wont to occur in a widely spread epidemic.

Yet, though the general proportion may not be much affected, still we are ready to admit that a case does now and then occur, where disease is shortly observed after the admittance of a sick person in a house or locality, and where the effect is so marked, so immediate and so general among those exposed, that we are compelled to admit that there is room for thinking, that the patient is somehow or other, in some degree at least, the occasion of the catastrophe.

It is sometimes observed that servant girls, affected with typhus fever, are in that state sent to their homes, and that disease shortly affects their brothers and sisters, but before such cases can be held as proving the existence of atmospheric contagion, there should be a strong assurance that the agencies of a most unwholesome character, known to exist in such cases, are inert, and that they which have on other occasions, without assistance, produced of themselves the distemper observed, have been altogether impotent and inactive.

Their case produces the usual effect, demands the exertion of night watching, spoken of already, as favourable to the accession of disease, and their house or apartment, close and confined as it usually is in that rank of life, becomes the abode of many unwholesome influences, and among others, of an atmosphere, deprived in a great degree of its more essential part, and loaded, too, with foreign gases, and even perhaps with chemical compounds of a virulent character, the products of putrefaction. If disease spreads much among those thus exposed, it seems fair to attribute the occurrence to these agencies known to be present, and known to be favourable to the production of sickness, and not to atmospheric contagion, as is almost universally done.

The case of disease appearing in a house previously healthy, after receiving one just recovered of disease, which it is by the way consonant with our experience to say, is much more rare than the other, or that of persons actually ill,—is occasionally noticed, and the explanation, perhaps, is, that the clothes may retain impurities acquired during the course of disease, and may on this occasion shew their activity.

CHAPTER IV.

There is no Evidence that Atmospheric Contagion Travels, or is Communicated from One Place to Another.

The question of the communication of atmospheric contagion from one place to another has almost universally, on occasions of pestilence, been much agitated, in respect to individual diseases, but seldom in a comprehensive way, embracing all diseases. We propose to inquire generally into the facts which are held to prove the principle of dissemination from one place to another—whether contagious atmosphere is transmitted from one country to another, from one town to another, and from hamlet to hamlet.

In the many works written by medical men on occasions of great epidemic disease, descriptive of the character of the prevalent distemper, there almost universally appear the most minute accounts of the route pursued by contagion, both fomitic and atmospheric, down to the noting of the very road, the very street or alley by which it reached a town—and of the manner in which it arrived, whether on the rags of a tattered beggar, or seated in a stage-coach.

The line of its progression is taken from the observation of disease, and from that alone. Wherever disease appears, there it is said that contagion has been carried or conveyed; and as a proof of that position, it is gravely maintained, that disease invariably breaks out where there are houses, and where communication is likely to be going on in some way or other. This most extraordinary fact proves what must certainly be thought not less extraordinary, that it appears in the abodes and habitations of men. But where else is disease, we would ask, to manifest itself, if among men at all, if not where alone they are to be found?—surely not among deserts uninhabitable, or on the frosty summit of an iceberg?

It is true that in the course of an epidemic, such as the

cholera, one country suffers before another; but there is no alternative to such a course if they are not to be simultaneously affected. And it signifies nothing that communication subsists between them. One part of a country, too, is ravaged first, then another, and so on—one town then another—one part of a town, and after it another part.

But it is evident, that if disease is to begin at all, it must begin somewhere, and if all parts are not to be seized on the same instant, that one will have precedence of another, and so on. Springing and propagating, from whatever causes, that character must hold, and surely it is wrong to hold a feature common to the effects of many causes as decisive evidence of the operation of one, and of one only.

The harvests of Europe begin in one country, sooner than in another. In many, harvest is earlier than in England, but it is never surmised that when that process begins in the latter country, that it is through the mediation of some such influence as contagion. It begins in England, too, it might be shewn, in places having communication with foreign countries. Nay, it might also be proven that the parts in which it in general commences are at the coast, where it is well known ships are wont to appear.

Were such an insane supposition made, the most obvious facts would necessarily be laid aside; but such gross blindness would not, we are satisfied, be much greater, than when the process of diseased action, marked out in an epidemic, is attributed to contagious atmosphere alone.

In the case of the harvest, it would argue a forgetfulness of the object held in view when the seed was sown,—in that of disease, an ignorance of the effects to be expected from the sowing of the seeds of pestilence (the exposure to the common epidemic influences alluded to above), in the first, an insensibility to the influence of climate, intensity of sun's rays, the quality of the soil, &c.:—And in the other, a blindness to the operation of circumstances not less potent, such as the time of application of the causes, the condition of the body, and the presence or absence of moral adjuvants.

It has universally held with all epidemic sickness, that parts of a country have been attacked in succession—that one town is visited after another, and one part of a town before another, whether the prevailing distemper have or have not been said to depend on contagion.

There is nothing extraordinary in the fact that all persons who are to suffer, do not become affected on one and the same day. Far from proving that any thing of the nature of contagion has been in operation, it only proves what may so readily be admitted, or at once readily understood, that all and sundry the inhabitants of a vast tract of country, inhabiting parts having different climates more or less mild, having different situations, some on the banks of rivers, some along the coast, some inland, some on boggy and some on dry soil; having different occupations, different houses, wearing different dresses, having different habits, different pursuits, different diet, different recreations, and perhaps having constitutions differing in aptitude to be acted upon, may not be all ready for the manifestation of disease on one and the same day, but may attain to that point at times corresponding with the operation of so many different circumstances.

In vegetation, which on the whole is much more simple than living animal organization, there is a gradation in the time at which its various individuals become ripe. The same grain is ripe in some districts weeks before it is ready in others, and even in the same farm, though the seed had been sown on the same day. Thus, by observing that the gradual development of disease over a country is the result of the varying activity and time of action of the epidemic influences, and perhaps of some condition of the body, varying in forwardness—it becomes unnecessary to have recourse to atmospheric contagion. It is unnecessary to repeat here what has been said relative to the operation of unwholesome agencies to account for the wide range of disease—over a country.

It is often said, as decisive proof of disease spreading by contagion, that a beggar, or some poor person left a town affected with disease, and entered another hitherto healthy—and that afterwards disease manifested itself there also.

In the first place, would not sickness have occurred notwithstanding? Its supporters say, not likely, when the effect followed, or immediately on the communication; but we reply, that communication took place before without any such immediate result, and that in all probability it had been going on freely all along, whatever regulation and hinderances might have been adopted.

It seems madness to think of stopping all communication with towns, in a free country such as this, where human intercourse is going on without interruption throughout the entire empire, or, indeed, anywhere at all, tolerably inhabited, or where commerce subsists.

It is in vain to endeavour to shew that opportunities for the transmission of contagious atmosphere have not occurred. The case involves an impossibility, for do not a thousand means of communication suggest themselves to the mind of the reader? The atmosphere itself, currents, winds, water, streams, &c.,—animals,—such as rats, mice, winged insects, &c. &c., which cannot be prevented from operating. We, therefore, leave this case, perhaps to the efforts of the advocates of quarantine regulations, who possibly may arrive at a happier result, and we proceed to the opposite case, where disease fails to spread, where communication does take place.

The advocates of contagion prove, where a disease appears in a town, that communication has taken place. That statement, as the reverse, can never be proven, is easily affirmed; and its insignificance corresponds with the facility with which it can be proven. Of course, it is obvious, that such a fact proves very little, either in reference to contagion or anything else.

We are prepared to prove, that communication has subsisted on many different occasions, without any unusual amount of sickness taking place. We know of many instances where disease has been prevailing in a town or village, which has failed to manifest itself in another at a short distance, although daily unrestrained communication was held.

At the end of the year 1835, and the beginning of the year 1836 the scarlet fever prevailed in Edinburgh to a great extent; and although great traffic was constantly going on between that town and Tranent, by means of foot-passengers, numerous carts and coaches, passing to and fro, daily, still that distemper failed to make its appearance in the latter town till the 20th of January, the day on which the first case was noticed.

That case did not occur at the point where the greatest thoroughfare subsists, but at one, the most remote from it.

Typhus fever has been prevailing, to a great extent, in Edinburgh, for many weeks past, but that disease has failed to make its appearance in Tranent (ten miles distant), although the road is constantly crowded with carriages, with vast numbers of carts conveying coals from that village to the capital, and with passengers both on horse and foot. It has not made its appearance, although several of the inhabitants of Tranent have lately lost relatives who have died of that disease, both in Edinburgh and Leith; and although a woman just recovered from that distemper, and come from the Royal Infirmary, has taken up her abode in this village.

Small-pox appeared about six weeks ago, simultaneously in two very filthy localities in Tranent, and it has been confined to them, although the most free communication has subsisted with other parts of the village, and it has failed to spread to the hamlets and farm-steadings around, notwithstanding the relatives of some of those labouring under that disease have travelled through the country, seeking charity.

We propose to close this part of the work. Much has been said in order to prove the position, that the doctrine of atmospheric contagion gains no support from the actual character of disease, no countenance from the ungarbled history of its career.

Arguments in favour of our views might have been drawn from the fact, that diseases said to be propagated by contagion, do not manifest themselves in all parts of the globe to which the poison would be likely to be taken, as they undoubtedly would do, were they dependent on the operation of one single object, such as contagious matter; and also from the consideration that those diseases, with whose causes we are intimately acquainted, by reason of their immediate operation, or of their being otherwise obvious, such as inflammation and wounds, are never said to be dependent on such an agency; but it is feared in the endeavour to be explicit, we have already been tiresome.

PART III

CHAPTER V

On Vitiated Air

The question of air holding in solution, an animal contagious matter, eliminated in the body of a sick person, and capable of producing the same disease, when inhaled by another, has hitherto occupied our attention.

It is now our design to treat of vitiated air, that is, an atmosphere deprived of part of its more essential principle, viz. oxygen gas, or tainted with the admixture of effluvia or gaseous products, from putrefying animal bodies, both living and dead, and from corrupting vegetable matter.

It is one of the most common, and most widely spread causes, of the most virulent and widely prevalent diseases, to which humanity is subject.

The importance of the atmosphere to the animal economy, is so very great, and its derangements so very hurtful to health, that it appears that a few observations respecting it may be useful to some non-professional readers. It may enable them to understand better the observations that are to follow on its vitiation.

The atmosphere is a fluid of an elastic nature, encompassing the globe, occupying the space comprehended from its surface, to the distance of twenty or thirty miles therefrom. It possesses weight, and it is by this property that water rises in pumps, and that mercury is sustained in the barometer. It is in constant motion, going, as it does, with the globe itself, revolving on its axis, and rushing, in counter streams, from the tropics to the poles, and from the poles to the tropics.

That portion nearest the sun becomes rarefied and lightened with the heat which it acquires:—it then rushes, by virtue of its comparative lightness, to the poles, and that in temperate regions presses forward to occupy its place.

By means of this motion, the temperature of the earth is kept pretty uniform, and it is corrected of any impure taint it may acquire.

The atmosphere is composed of two gases, oxygen and nitrogen, a small quantity of watery vapour, and a fraction of carbonic acid gas, or fixed air.

Oxygen is the agent on which its more active properties depend. The other component, viz. nitrogen, serving to dilute it.

They are united in the proportion of about seventy-seven of nitrogen by volume, and twenty-one of oxygen, the rest being made up of watery vapour, and carbonic acid gas.

The atmosphere supports combustion,—oxygen gas being the essential agent. During combustion, it is consumed, and at the end of the process, it will be found wanting,—the other gas being undiminished.

This may be seen, at least the diminution in the volume of air, by burning a candle in a large wide mouthed bottle, inverted over coloured water. As it continues to burn, the water ascends in the bottle, and occupies the place of the oxygen consumed.

Atmospheric air supports respiration, a process essential to the continuance of life. Oxygen gas here, too, is the agent on which it depends. Air, which has been once respired, is found to be deprived of part of its oxygen, from ten to twelve per cent.

Air, deprived of oxygen, or even deprived of a small portion of it, is unfit for respiration. A mouse, put into a vessel containing air, which has been robbed of that fluid, dies immediately. Put into one containing pure air, it breathes well at first, but, as the oxygen gets less, its breathing becomes laboured, it is convulsed, and shortly dies.

The air is concerned, besides, in a thousand operations, constantly going on at the surface of the earth. It gives up a portion of its component parts in an immense number, and in a considerable proportion receives bodies foreign to its constitution.

By one set of operations, it is deprived of its oxygen, and becomes vitiated by the admixture of deleterious principles. By others, again, its oxygen is restored, and the impurities removed; so that between two opposite forces, it is in general kept in a wholesome condition.

An immense number of bodies on the surface of the earth, are constantly attracting to themselves the oxygen of the air; some become what is called oxydized, as the metals, the dull incrustation which is found upon them after long exposure to the air, being an oxide, or a combination of the metal, and the oxygen of the air. Some bodies become acids, as the various vegetable juices which form their respective acids, by combination with the oxygen of the atmosphere.

During fermentation, the oxygen is absorbed, and carbonic acid is evolved. During putrefaction, oxygen is taken up also. There are many operations, too, connected with the arts, in which that fluid is abstracted from the air. The very soil is constantly acting on the atmosphere, and is, indeed, one vast and extended laboratory, where chemical processes, on a large scale, are going on without interruption. The putrefaction of the animal and vegetable materials, used as manure, is much promoted by free exposure to the air; hence one of the advantages of ploughing the land so universally adopted. The very nature of the soil is greatly altered by that process, and much of that change depends not only on the chemical processes just spoken of, but upon the action of the air itself, on the essential particles of the clod. From the surface of newly turned up soil, it is understood by intelligent agriculturists, that much gaseous or elastic vapour is evolved; and we have heard it observed by intelligent ploughmen, that one of the most delightful things is the air which arises from newly ploughed fields in the morning. It is said that it imparts an invigorating, and wholesome sensation throughout the body, and from thence to the mind.

All those processes we referred to, abstract from the atmosphere its most essential part, the oxygen gas. Did that process of abstraction go on without its being counterbalanced by others, imparting that principle to supply the place of that abstracted, then the atmosphere in the course of time would become unfit to support combustion or flame,—unfit to support animal respiration; and the consequence would be, that the surface of the earth would soon be uninhabitable, would soon be a lifeless desert. Such would be the inevitable consequence.

But a wise and a good Creator has prevented the occurrence of that catastrophe. He has so ordered it, that one department of nature shall correct the bad tendencies of the other;—he has placed a weight at the opposite end of the balance, to counterpoise and balance the glorious work of his hand. Animal life is met by vegetable life: their results are made to neutralize those of each other, and with a wisdom truly the Father's, found in his works alone, he has made the apparently hurtful consequence of animal life, the very means for the maintenance of the life of vegetation. The results of the function of respiration so necessary to animals, are highly useful to vegetables. Those products that are hurtful are absorbed by the leaves of plants, which are analogous to our lungs or breathing apparatus, and the oxygen consumed by animals is replaced by the evolution of a large quantity of that principle.

During sunshine, plants, especially in water, give out a large quantity of that principle, as may be seen by putting grass leaves into a jar filled with water, and exposing them to sunshine. Bubbles of air soon appear, and collect at the top of the jar; they are oxygen gas.

The evolution of oxygen gas in sunshine, is the chief means with which we are acquainted, by which the chemical equipoise of the atmosphere is maintained, against the operations constantly going on, to which we alluded.

These observations relate to the chemical composition of the air, considered as one great whole.

There are many situations in which it becomes not only deprived of its oxygen in part, but becomes vitiated by admixture with foreign bodies or vapours, most detrimental to health, in short, most pestiferous. But, before pointing out the manner in which it becomes so tainted, and its unwholesome consequences, we would here point out the use of the atmosphere. By the act of respiration, air is carried into the lungs; it acts upon the blood brought there in large quantities, and spread out in innumerable vessels, forming a sort of network. The blood, upon its arrival at the lungs, is dark, grumous, and unfit for the maintenance of life, and the nutrition of the body; but, under the action of the air, it becomes florid or crimson, has changes wrought upon it, by which it is fitted to perform its various and important functions.

This chemical process gives a crimson and florid hue to the old blood of the system, and imparts a colour and other qualities to the fluid brought from the bowels, the result of digestion, which give it the character of blood. It gives to that fluid the last preparation before being converted into blood.

The heat of the body, which is above that of the surrounding atmosphere, is maintained by the chemical changes which occur between the mass of blood in the lungs, and the air to which it is there exposed. There is a constant generation of heat, which is diffused along with the blood throughout the whole system,—to supply the place of that which is ever being abstracted by surrounding bodies, among which exists a constant tendency to preserve an equilibrium of temperature.

When the atmosphere is vitiated, it is reasonable to suppose, that the changes in the blood passing through the lungs will not take place in their wonted integrity, and that, among other results, a diminution of the vital heat of the body may be experienced.

Vitiated air admits of division into different kinds:—

1st, Into air simply deprived more or less of its oxygen.

2d, Into air holding in solution, or having mingled with it, effluvia from animal bodies, living and dead.

3d, Into air holding in solution, or having mingled with it, noxious gases or effluvia arising from decomposing vegetable matter.

Vitiated air, of every kind, is unwholesome and favourable to the invasion of disease.

Vitiated air has been coexistent with many of the most appalling visitations of disease, which have befallen man since the creation of the world. It delights in the production of the most formidable distempers, such as are marked with extreme debility and proneness to the putrefactive character.

The plague, in its various visitations, from the time of its prevalence in Athens, as described by Thucydides and Lucretius, down to the period when it last raged in England, viz. in the year 1665, has been observed to be coincident, for the most part, with circumstances proving the existence of vitiated air: and at this day the most mortal diseases prevail, where foul air exists, whether that arises from this or that source.

The atmosphere becomes vitiated, when great numbers of men in health are crowded together in apartments too close and confined to admit of a sufficient supply of pure air for the perfect maintenance of respiration. In this case, the vitiation is effected by the abstraction of the oxygen of the atmosphere, the exhalation of carbonic acid gas, and the dissemination of effluvia which arise from the bodies of those who are confined.

The immediate effects of confinement to an atmosphere thus vitiated are, oppressed breathing, sense of great anxiety and suffering, fixedness of the eyes, and torpor, which gradually increases to insensibility; and the miserable sufferer dies bereft of sense and motion, from suffocation.

When the atmosphere is not so impure as to cause immediate death, disease of a putrid character, for the most part takes place. Typhus fever attacked those persons who survived the memorable struggle in the black hole of Calcutta.

A low form of fever used to commit great havoc in jails and other places of confinement, where prisoners were wont to be crowded together in great numbers, from the atmosphere being deprived of its more vital part, and being loaded with unwholesome emanations arising from the filthy persons, and clothes of those confined.

This disease is called "Jail Fever," and manifests a peculiarly malignant character.

In hospitals crowded with wounded soldiers, but otherwise in health, where sufficient ventilation cannot be maintained, the same distemper makes its appearance, and is there denominated "Hospital Fever."

In besieged towns and in camps, where the inmates are exposed to the offensive and unwholesome effluvia, commonly experienced in such situations, the same putrid disease prevails, and goes under the name of "Camp Fever."

Air Vitiated With Effluvia From Bodies In A State Of Disease.

Air vitiated with effluvia from bodies in a state of disease, and their excretions, has been variously denominated.

By some it has been styled "Contagious Air;" by some "Infectious Air;" and, when it is in connection with fever, "Febrile Miasm or Contagion."

Vitiated air of this kind differs from that referred to above, in this particular, that it arises from bodies in a state of disease.

Both forms of vitiated air produce, or assist to produce, disease of the same character; but as the latter form not only goes to produce disease, but arises from disease also, it has been considered to be analogous to the contagious poisons, such as those of small-pox, cow-pox, and the like.

From the circumstance of this vitiated air arising from persons in disease, and assisting in the propagation of the same malady, it has all along been regarded as a specific contagious animal poison in an atmospheric menstruum; and thus has been created the perplexing and entangled web of confusion and vagueness that has been wove around the principles, viz. contagious poisons, and vitiated air arising from effluvia from persons in disease, and from their excretions.

From this circumstance, these principles, viz. specific contagious poisons, and vitiated air arising from persons in disease, have been erroneously classed together, and a supposed analogy has been created.

But these principles are widely different in their nature, and in the laws by which they are regulated.

The specific contagious poisons produce the same diseases as those with which the bodies, whence they arose, were affected, and them only; and their operation is marked by uniform effects, observing stated and unvarying periods. Vitiated air, of the kind under examination, though it arises from persons in a state of disease, and is sometimes known to operate in the production or propagation of the same distemper, does not always induce disease, does not induce that disease only, whence it sprung, but various others; and, in short, its effects are not uniform, and do not observe stated and unvarying periods.

The specific contagious poisons produce their peculiar diseases, as their proper and only effects, without the cooperation of other influences; but vitiated air, when the same disease extends, whence it arose, cannot be said to be causing its proper, only, and peculiar effects, as the same disease does not invariably follow its action. In general, the effluvia which proceed from a sick person, where they prove hurtful, cause the same distemper as that with which he is affected; for instance, the effluvia arising from a person affected with typhus fever, produce that disease again:—but that is not always the case, and an instance will be presently detailed, where the effluvia which proceeded from a body dead of one disease, produced another of a very different nature.

The reason that the presence of vitiated air is generally attended with the same disease as that with which the body is affected, whence it sprung, is, that there is existing at the time, a disposition to that particular malady: and the vitiated air only gives it form by acting as an ordinary exciting cause upon individuals prepared for its invasion.

It appears probable that vitiated air, unlike the palpable contagious poisons, assists in the production of that disease only which is prevailing, or to which there exists a disposition from the operation of other agencies; and it appears probable that vitiated air, whether it arises from persons affected with this or that disease, will, within certain limits, produce one disease as readily as another, the required particular disposition being present; for instance, that the effluvia from a small-pox patient will induce small-pox or typhus fever, according as there exists a disposition to the one disease or the other, and *vice versa*.

The effluvia arising from newly opened graves have been often productive of putrid fever.

The following case will shew that effluvia arising from the remains of a person who died of consumption of the lungs, and not of small-pox, produced that disease, viz. small-pox. When that case occurred, small-pox was prevailing, and doubtless, had there been existing at the time a disposition to putrid fever, that disease, and not small-pox, would have been induced by the effluvia which arose from the grave.

In September 1834, Peter Macawley, about twenty-eight years of age, gardener and grave-digger, was employed in the churchyard of Tranent. While busily digging a grave, he unexpectedly struck a coffin with his spade, and broke it open. The coffin contained the remains of an old woman, who had died of consumption of the lungs, and who had been interred about fourteen months.

There immediately issued from the coffin the most offensive effluvia, which threatened suffocation, and made him feel very unwell.

He proceeded home, and continued throughout the night very poorly, giddy, and uncomfortable. He rose next morning, and although no better, proceeded to the churchyard, gave some directions, and returned home, feeling giddy and unsteady. He was put to bed, and passed a very uncomfortable night.

Called in next morning to prescribe for him, I found him to be affected with severe pain of head, great heat and sweating of skin, and great quickness of pulse. He complained of thirst, could take no food, and was occasionally delirious. On the third day of his illness, pimples appeared over the whole surface of the body, which gradually becoming larger, assumed the form of small-pox. The pocks or pustules did not mature or fill with matter in the usual way, but continued throughout to be flat, and assumed a dark blue or inky colour.

His strength fast declined,—he became very low,—muttered incoherently to himself, and symptoms of a putrid character supervening, and the energies of the system fast failing, he died insensible about the twelfth day of his illness, of the worst form of immature, putrid, confluent small-pox I had ever witnessed.

He was a powerful, well-formed, and laborious man, was in good general health up to the moment of his being affected in the grave,—and it was not ascertained that he had been in a situation to receive infection from any other source.

Vitiated air arising from persons in a state of disease, is found in those situations only where the apartment is close and confined, where the person and clothes are allowed to remain in a state of impurity, where the secretions and excretions are left to ferment; and, in short, where no attention is paid to cleanliness, the removal of respired air, and the introduction of a fresh atmosphere. The production of vitiated air is thus only occasional, while, in the contagious diseases, the specific poisons are produced in every case of their respective diseases, and were they capable of being diffused in the atmosphere, there would be present as constantly an atmospheric contagion.

When vitiated air is produced, its removal can readily be accomplished, as daily experience, and the testimony of Dr Haygarth, given at the beginning of this work, amply prove.

Air Vitiated With Effluvia From Dead Animal Matter.

There is still another source whence effluvia of a pestiferous nature arise. Dead animal matter, during putrefaction, exhales gases which taint the atmosphere, and render it unwholesome.

When these materials are exposed to heat and moisture, the decomposition is rapid, and the air becomes more obviously tainted than when that process is retarded by cold, breezy weather, and some other circumstances. When the decomposition takes place in the open air, and when that is kept in motion, the quantity of decomposing materials not being very great, the bad effects are not so serious.

When, however, buried along with a sufficient quantity of atmospheric air, to allow of the play of the chemical affinities, and kept there a considerable time, if they be exhumed previous to their total digestion or complete assimilation with surrounding objects, effluvia are exhaled, having the most intolerable stench, causing instant sickness, faintness, and giddiness, and eventually producing disease.

"Thus, we are told by Fourcroy, that in some of the burial-grounds of France, whose graves are dug up sooner than they ought to be, the effluvium from an abdomen, (belly), suddenly opened by the stroke of the mattock, strikes so forcibly upon the grave-digger, as to throw him into a state of asphyxy, if close at hand; and if at a little distance, to oppress him with vertigo, fainting, nausea, loss of appetite, and tremors for many hours: whilst numbers of those who live in the neighbourhood of such cemeteries labour under dejected spirits, sallow countenances, and febrile emaciation."[5]

Instances are likewise known where graves containing human bodies, long dead of plague, upon being opened, have emitted effluvia, which have produced typhus fever among the workmen.

It is probable that, in general, the effluvia arising from dead animal materials, undergoing decomposition in the ordinary way, are the common results of the putrefactive fermentation,—carbonic acid gas, hydrogen, nitrogen, &c.

These gases form various combinations; carbonic acid gas and hydrogen gas forming carburetted hydrogen, an inflammable gas, the same as is used for the purpose of illumination, and which cannot support respiration. Hydrogen unites with nitrogen, and forms ammonia, or spirit of hartshorn, which is volatile, and imparts a strong odour to the atmosphere, such as is experienced in stables and byres, producing sneezing and watering of the eyes.

Hydrogen, at its extrication, sometimes carries with it a portion of phosphorus, already contained in the decomposing body, and becomes phosphuretted hydrogen, a gas which ignites spontaneously in the atmosphere, the same that is sometimes observed in churchyards under the title of corpse-lights.

Hydrogen sometimes also unites with sulphur, and the combination is called sulphuretted hydrogen, a gas readily discovered by its offensive odour,—which it imparts to many very useful mineral waters.

These gases are discovered, not only in an atmosphere exposed to decomposing dead animal materials, but are also found in that atmosphere containing numbers of men in health, closely crowded together, and persons suffering putrid diseases, where no attention is paid to cleanliness and the removal of impurities.

A body affected with putrid disease is more liable to decomposition than one in health; and the secretions and excretions are more prone to putrefaction, and the emission of effluvia or gases.

---

[5] Good's Study of Medicine, vol. ii. page 65.

Some facts are known, which shew that bodies, in some forms of low or malignant disease, both before and after death, possess a virulence, never found in bodies in health, or affected with disease of a non-malignant character. The worst consequences have followed wounds in the dissection of bodies recently dead of typhus fever; the introduction, under the skin, of the fluid contained in the petechiæ or black spots common in that disease, and even the washing of bandages and clothes employed in cases of mortification and the like.

In such diseases, the body becomes a very centre of contamination and virulence; its fluids become acrid and poisonous; and on the surface of the body, fluids are elaborated, which are productive of the most malignant and pestiferous effects. Whether these fluids, those virulent secretions, are ever diffused in the air, and impart to it their deadly properties, is a point of much interest, but one which cannot be entertained here.

CHAPTER VI

Air Vitiated by Admixture with Effluvia Arising from the Decomposition of Vegetable Matter on the Surface of the Earth

It is not only from such sources as those already treated of, that effluvia or gases arise, to contaminate the atmosphere, and to spread disease among men and beasts. Effluvia likewise spring from the putrefaction of vegetables; and, in many instances, from circumstances favourable to their development and action, they so vitiate the atmosphere, that its respiration induces some of the most virulent diseases, and, where the effects are not so serious, a state of slow sickness and great suffering is often the lot of the sufferer, during the whole course of his miserable existence. The situations of these effluvia will shortly be pointed out, along with the respective diseases incident to them.

But let us for a moment consider the changes on which these effluvia depend. Putrefaction of vegetable matter is one of the many wise provisions which the Almighty has instituted for the accomplishment of his comprehensive plan of the creation.

The surface of the earth is covered with vegetation, to supply man with food, and likewise to support the various animals placed below him in the scale of creation, so necessary to his comfort and existence. They are consumed, and, by means of digestion, become component parts of animals; and when these, in their turn, die, they go down to the earth, whence they originally sprung.

Mixed there, with other matters composing the soil, the carcasses of animals afford nourishment to vegetation again, and once more they are found as the component principles of vegetable forms. Thus the animal is constantly supplying food to the vegetable world, which, in its turn, supplies food to the other again.

In life, we found them performing functions useful to each other, and mutually correcting their unwholesome effects; in death, they are no less useful: the one is converted into the other.

All animated creation is the scene of endless changes, and is the object of successive transformations. 'Tis one mighty circle, of a thousand parts, constantly revolving,—one part occupying now this, now that place,—and each taking the place of that next it, till at length it completes the entire circle; and even then the race is not yet run, the revolution must be performed again and again, to the very end of time.

The immediate agency by which these wonderful changes are effected, is putrefaction. We have alluded to it shortly, in connection with man in health, in disease, and in death.

We have now to speak of putrefaction in connection with dead vegetable matter, in marshy situations, &c., where it is the occasion of much disease.

There is no reason to believe that it was the design of the Almighty, that the process of putrefaction, which is so essential to the great plan of successive races of animals and vegetables, should be the active engine of pestilence, which it is in many situations.

That is not the necessary consequence of putrefaction; and when it does occur, it is rather the effect of accidental circumstances. Under ordinary circumstances, where putrefaction goes on, as among vegetables moderately moist, exposed to currents of air, and mixed up with the soil, as in the various processes of agriculture, no bad results are experienced.

But when vegetation is allowed to go on year after year, without being cropped, where, as it ripens, it withers and dies; and when it dies, is allowed to accumulate and putrefy, where there is much moisture, much solar heat, and little motion of the air, where, perhaps, other circumstances are operating, favourable to rapid decomposition, effluvia are wont to ascend and vitiate the atmosphere.

Such a vitiated atmosphere has acquired various appellations, according to the place in which it has been observed, and according to the effects or diseases it produces.

But, under whatever name it passes, its origin is the same, namely, decomposing vegetable matter on the surface of the earth, perhaps, in some situations, mixed more or less with dead animal matter.

It is decomposing vegetable matter which produces the yellow fever of the West Indies, the jungle fever of India, the deadly pestilential fever of the coast of Africa, the ague in this country and in many others, the cretinism of Switzerland, the pellagra of Milan, the unwholesome condition of humanity in many parts of Italy, and especially in the country surrounding Rome, or the Campagna of Rome, as it is called. The decomposition, however, takes place under circumstances somewhat different, and hence the difference in the results of its action.

These effects are attributed to the decomposition of vegetable matter; but there is room to think that, along with that, there is combined no very insignificant proportion of matter of an animal nature.

It may safely be inferred, that wherever there is vegetation, there animals are found also; and it is well known that vast numbers of many kinds of animals live wherever decomposition is taking place, especially if the situation is warm and sheltered. The carcasses of these animals will be added to the vegetable matter, and add to the common mass of corruption.

That matter in swamps, and in unwholesome situations, said to be purely vegetable, is then a compound of animal and vegetable origin; and these effluvia arise, not from vegetable decomposition only, but from both dead animal and vegetable substances in a state of putrefaction.

There is little known of the composition of these effluvia. We are most conversant with their situations, and their effects upon health. In different situations, they produce different diseases. But no known facts entitle us positively to say that their composition is different. It is a remarkable fact, but one well ascertained, that the atmosphere, in all parts of the world, in all climates, and in all situations, is much the same in its chemical composition. It manifests the same general physical characters in all situations, whether healthy or pestilential, and the nicest investigations have detected nothing in an atmosphere known to be pestilential, that is not found in the most wholesome.

However, there is much reason to think, that this circumstance is owing, not to the absence of hurtful gases, but to the comparative insignificance of their volume beside that of the atmosphere itself, so vast in its dimensions.

Medical men have been disposed to think that effluvia which cause one disease, say the yellow fever, are not the same as that which cause another, say the fever of the coast of Africa. The only reason offered is the difference of the diseases; but that is not enough to prove that the effluvia are different in their nature. Different effects, or effects so modified as to appear very different, are the results of the same cause on many occasions. The smoke of tobacco will make one person feel comfortable, another merry, another sick, another faint, and so on; but it would be unfair, from these differences in the effects, to pronounce that tobacco-smoke was in all these cases different in its own nature.

We are satisfied that the effluvia or gases arising from marshy or unwholesome soil, are the same, generally speaking, in all situations, whatever disease is produced; and that the difference in the results is to be attributed to the varying circumstances under which they act,—for instance, the constancy or inconstancy of their operation, their greater or less intensity, the greater or less degree of concomitant moisture and heat, the greater or less amount of motion of the air,—the sheltered situation of human habitations,—the condition of the body, its predispositions from native country and the like, and the individual being accustomed or unaccustomed to the action of effluvia.

Gases are known to arise from the marshy grounds mentioned, where animal and vegetable matter is putrefying, from the fact, that the neighbourhood of swamps is most unwholesome, the inhabitants and visitors almost uniformly suffering, because unwholesome effluvia are invariably known to emanate where animal and vegetable matter is thus corrupting, and because the gases themselves may be seen rising in bubbles out of putrid water, containing dead animal and vegetable matter in a state of corruption.

These bubbles contain gases the very same as are disengaged when animal and vegetable matter are putrefying among water. They are nearly the same as proceed from merely animal matter dead and putrefying, not incorporated with the soil, viz. carburetted hydrogen, or inflammable gas, carbonic acid gas, or fixed air, and sometimes a little phosphuretted and likewise sulphuretted hydrogen.

These gases are sometimes appreciable to the organ of smell. Carburetted hydrogen is very strong, and is perceptible in many situations where there is much corruption going on; for instance, at the meadow-ground between the Dairy, on the Portobello road, and Comely Green, near Edinburgh, where the stench is so strong as to prove most offensive to passengers on the road. The source is the corrupting animal and vegetable materials, in the foul water conducted from Edinburgh, and made to overflow the ground, for the purposes of irrigation.

In such situations, it is not uncommon to observe lights floating along during the night, and superstition has not failed to make them represent evil spirits. They are known by the name of "Will o' Wisp" and "Jack o' Lantern;" and have, on many occasions, proved objects of no slight dread to many ignorant persons. The lights are merely ignited carburetted hydrogen gas,—the same kind of gas as that used for lighting our shops and houses.

The gas is ignited, perhaps, by the rising to the surface of the putrid water, of a bubble of phosphuretted hydrogen, which, as was before observed, burns the moment it comes in contact with the atmosphere.

Other products of an aeriform kind may be evolved also, but we have no direct evidence of their existence,—but an atmosphere, loaded with vapours of the kind mentioned, is enough to account for the production of the observed disease, in all its varied forms, when there is conjoined with it other unwholesome agencies. In some countries, the pestilential air is present throughout the year, for instance, in the country around Rome, in the fens of Lincolnshire, where ague is seldom absent; in others it is periodical, chiefly confined to the hot and rainy seasons, as in India and in the West Indies, where fevers prevail to a great extent; and in others, again, it is observed only when the wind blows from a particular direction.

These effluvia are conveyed to a distance by currents, and produce their peculiar effects, more or less, upon almost all they encounter. The malaria at Rome is carried by the wind into the city, by the channels most open to its entrance; and those parts, it is said by medical men who reside there, that are most exposed to the wind blowing off the adjacent marshy grounds, are most unhealthy. It is for that reason that the suburbs are more unwholesome than the interior of that city, where the wind does not find ready access, on account of the obstacles offered to its course by the high buildings. The high houses and streets thus act as a barrier against the entrance of the pestilence, and it is even said that the narrowest streets there, are the most healthy, as they shut out the pestilential vapour.

An obstacle of the same kind is offered by hills which interrupt the course of winds carrying with them vapours from marshy grounds. In the West Indies, where the yellow fever commits such frightful ravages, many instances are known where a town or district retains its health, from the shelter which a hill affords against the visitation of a wind that has loaded itself with deadly miasms, while sweeping over a marsh or swamp. It is the practice of those residing in those countries, not only to remove from the swamps, but also from those points to which the wind blows after passing over them.

Inattention to that consideration has led to the loss of much human life, and to the fruitless expenditure of much money in the erection of houses, barracks, and the like, which, after completion, have been found to be totally uninhabitable, from the pestilential vapours carried to them by the winds. In illustration of the influence of winds, we submit the following interesting extract from Dr Good's Study of Medicine. He has been speaking of effluvia from animal matter. "But the foul and stinking Harmattan," (a pestilential wind) "when it rushes from the south-east upon the Guinea coast, loaded with vegetable exhalations alone, with which it impregnates itself while sweeping over the immense uninhabitable swamps and oozy mangrove thickets of the sultry regions of Benin, triumphs in a still more rapid and wasteful destruction; so much that Dr Lind informs us, that the mortality produced by this pestilential vapour in the year 1754 or 1755 was so general, that in several negro towns, the living were not sufficient to bury the dead; and that the gates of Cape Coast Castle were shut up for want of sentinels to perform duty. Blacks and whites falling promiscuously before this fatal scourge."

So loaded is the air on some occasions with these pestilential vapours, that they attach themselves to whatever objects they meet, houses, the sides of hills, and woods, through which they pass along with the wind, and so completely has a wood stripped the currents of their baneful accompaniments, that they have been respired after with no injury whatever.

Trees are found to give great shelter and salubrity to towns in this way, acting as they do as so many sieves retaining impurities.

It is understood that the effluvia arising from putrefying vegetable matters ascend high in the atmosphere under the influence of the solar rays, and spread far and wide, and that at night during the cold they fall with the dew to the ground again, and impart to it and to those exposed to its action, much virulence. The ground is there known to be extremely unwholesome, and those who have been compelled by want, by sickness, while travelling, overtaking them, or by being benighted, to lie down with nothing but the soil for a couch, and with no shelter from the vapours and dew that falls at night, save the sky itself, have felt this pestilential influence: on the morrow they awake distressed, parched, and affected with headach, and the usual symptoms of malignant fever.

With the close of day or the setting of the sun, the pestilential vapour falls and envelopes the country and the habitations of men with a deadly mantle—and it is then unsafe to venture into the open air in many of the finest countries of the world.

The pestilential effects of exposure to these night dews and vapours have, on many occasions, been experienced by soldiers encamping in the open grounds, and our gallant countrymen on foreign service are wont to yield in fearful numbers to a foe, merciless and unsparing.

But it is not in swampy grounds only that these vapours arise, for there is reason to think that in those places where sickness is constant, and where no such dampness of ground is observed, that decomposition of animal and vegetable matter is going on some depth below the surface, and that the extricated gases issue through the soil. This is rendered almost certain, by the fact which has sometimes been observed, that the most dangerous and sickly season is, when the ground is parched and rent with heat, permitting the exhalations generated below to ascend into the atmosphere. Instances of this occurred among our soldiers in the Peninsular war—the season, marked with the greatest prevalence of disease, the common result of vitiated air, being that when the soil was most rent with heat.

In some parts of Italy, it is remarked by that eminent physician and philosopher, Dr James Johnstone, in his admirable volume, entitled the Diary of a Philosopher, which, by the way, is a work of rare virtue, in so much as it is replete, not only with accurate medical knowledge, but with reflections in literature and the fine arts such as prove an intimacy with polite learning not always found, that fever and that general unwholesome state of body, observed in districts infested with vitiated air, prevail where inquiry has discovered no appearance of unusual dampness and corruption of the soil. He thinks that streams of putrid water, containing animal and vegetable materials, that have sunk down from the surface, in some part of their course are making their way at a little depth, and that when the soil, parched with excessive heat and drought, becomes rent, as it commonly does, the emanations previously confined rush out by the channels now presented by these fissures, and deal their deadly effects around.

Such an explanation seems to me highly probable, and deserving of more inquiry. Connected with this subject, the following facts may be interesting, and assist in forming an estimate of the probability of the truth of that explanation.

In mines, as well as on the surface of the earth, changes are constantly going on; and as in the latter situation the animal, vegetable, and mineral components of the soil are decomposing, so the minerals in the former are giving out some of their component parts and abstracting oxygen, &c. in turn from the atmosphere.

In mines some of the fossils attract oxygen from the air, but the chief process by which the atmosphere becomes vitiated there, is by the evolution of gases from the minerals. In coal pits the principal gases emitted are carbonic acid gas, commonly known as fixed air, which will support neither animal life nor combustion, as proved by the disastrous results on men having been confined in it, and by the extinction of light when immersed therein, and carburetted hydrogen gas, known as fire-damp, which cannot support respiration, and which takes fire when brought in contact with a light. These gases are the results of chemical changes going on in the minerals, in the same way as the gases before alluded to attend the decomposition of animal and vegetable substances.

These gases arise not only from the minerals exposed to view at the various surfaces, as the roof, sides, and pavement of coal pits, but issue also from the unworked minerals in the interior, by fissures or cracks in the various strata, produced by the violence used in detaching the minerals.

These fissures extend in the course of the beds, or strata, and are often scarcely visible, but are sometimes so wide as to admit the finger. It is probable that they sometimes extend a considerable way into the solid minerals.

In general, from these fissures there is constantly issuing streams of gas, of a nature varying with the character of the minerals, but for the most part they are such as have been mentioned. In the mines of Great Britain, when the atmosphere above is much agitated, as by the prevalence of southerly winds, and more especially if the violence amounts to what is termed a storm, the gases pour out in prodigious quantities, making a rushing noise, and filling the pit and excavated parts. The pit then becomes so full as to interfere with the operations of the men, who are frequently, for their safety, obliged to retire. In this case the atmosphere is lightened, and the pressure it is constantly exerting on all bodies with which it comes in contact is diminished, and the consequence is, that the gases rush out, under the circumstances already mentioned. It is known, that, during the prevalence of stormy weather, the mercury in a barometer falls; it is for a like reason, the weight upon it being less. Not only the gases issue from their caverns when the air is thus lightened, but water contained in fissures in the floor or pavement of mines rises also, sometimes to the amount of an inch or two, and it is no uncommon thing to see the extrication of vapour from a little collection of water on the floor, such as takes place when water is boiling, a movement which it very much resembles.

These facts shew that it is not improbable that pestilential vapours, ordinarily passing under the soil, may be extricated when fissures are present. It may happen that effluvia may be prevented from issuing even when fissures exist in the soil, from an increase in the weight of the atmosphere, and in this way may be explained the occasional disappearance of pestilence with a change of weather, not unfrequently remarked in some tropical countries.

During the prevalence of strong north, north-east, and north-west winds, blowing with considerable violence the currents in mines are reversed—for, instead of gases issuing from the fissures and crannies, currents of atmospheric air pour into them. These currents may be felt with the hand, and the ear can detect the rushing sound; a flame applied to a fissure is immediately drawn in, shewing the direction of the current. These facts illustrate the influence which the state of the atmosphere has upon terrestrial vapours.

As has been already observed, the exhalations from the soil obtain different names from the effects they are wont to produce. When they produce intermittent fever or ague, they are termed marsh miasms. When they produce the various forms of malignant fever, such as the yellow, the bilious fever of India, and the coast of Africa, simply pestilential effluvia—and when they induce general bad health and degeneracy of the inhabitants of a country, they are styled malaria, an Italian expression signifying bad air.

As the subject appears one which may interest the general reader, it is proposed to add a few observations on the diseases which are caused by air vitiated with effluvia from the soil.

CHAPTER VII

Malignant Fever

A vast proportion of the most virulent diseases to which the human race is subject in almost all parts of the world, but more especially in tropical regions, is produced by the action of effluvia arising from decomposing dead animal and vegetable matter on the surface of the earth, and incorporated with the soil. These effluvia are the immediate instrument by which thousands of our fellow men are annually deprived of existence, the career of the young and the robust is abruptly stopped, never again to be renewed. Malignant fever is the disease, by which death is occasioned from these effluvia; and this fever assumes forms, characters, and titles, various and manifold. It ravages in almost every country within the tropics, and in many situations it annually commits the most dreadful havoc—cutting down so rapidly that the ordinary forms of burial cannot be observed. Whole communities suffer, the inhabitants of a particular tract of country are sometimes almost extirpated, and to visit some countries is almost to incur death from pestilence, so near to certain is attack, and its destructive character is so uniform.

The average duration of life in many countries is extremely low, chiefly on account of the wasteful career of that scourge, under its various characters and designations; and it is not saying too much that there the number of deaths is four times as great as occurs in our own happy country.

In those regions in which malignant fever prevails so much, almost every inhabitant at one period of his life, sooner or later, is afflicted with it. If he survive he is more fortunate than thousands of those who lived beside him; but his health is often deteriorated, he is often deprived of that vigour and elasticity both of mind and body, which spring from a sound constitution, and he not unfrequently lingers under the sufferings of chronic disease till his life is gradually though slowly exhausted; unless, indeed, as often happens, it is suddenly terminated by a fresh attack of the active pestilence.

"Almost every territory in which it (malignant fever) has committed its ravages has given it a new name. It is as gorgeously arrayed with titles as the mightiest monarch of the East. From the depredations it has committed in the West Indies, and on the American coast, it has been called the St Domingo, Barbadoes, Jamaica, and American fever; and from its fatal visitations on the Guinea Coast, and its adjoining islands, the Bulam fever. In British India it is distinguished by the name of Jungle fever, and still farther to the east by that of Mal de Siam. Nearer home, in the lowlands of Hungary, and along the south of Spain, it is called the Hungarian or the Andalusian pestilence. From its rapid attack on ships' crews, that are fresh to its influence, the French denominate it Fievre Matelotte, (fever of sailors) as the Spanish and Portuguese call it vomito Prieto or black vomit, from the slaty or purplish and granular suburra (grounds) thrown up from the stomach in the last stage of the disease; while, as its ordinary source is moist lands, it has frequently been named Paludal Fever."[6]

This fever is severe with new settlers in these countries. Persons visiting places in which it is endemic, during its severity almost necessarily suffer, but sometimes they escape with a slight attack, in which case they are said to have had a "seasoning fever." The pestilential vapours may be carried to a great distance, by winds and currents. Instances have already been given where districts are immediately rendered unhealthy upon the visitation of a wind which has passed over an unhealthy swamp at a distance. Many instances are also well known where ships, riding at the distance of a league from an unhealthy coast, have had their crews affected with the distemper, on the vapours being sent among them by the wind coming off that direction. The British navy is, alas, too familiar with instances of ships being visited by that pestilence when lying off the coast of Africa, where, too, no direct communication had been maintained. The most appalling mortality occurs in these cases; it is not unusual

[6] Good's Study of Medicine, vol. ii. p. 145.

during the short period a ship remains on that station for the whole officers and crew to be swept away in one general tide of death, and it not unfrequently happens that, after the short space of three years, the ordinary time of service, that when a ship returns to England, she has not a hand on board she carried out—but is manned with a crew that has succeeded one which had, in its turn, taken the place of that which danced in joy, and looked all gallantry, only a few short months before, when with hearty huzzas they left their native land, and committed themselves to their bark and to the buoyant billows. At the time of the expedition to Walcheren a disastrous state of health prevailed among the soldiery in Holland, in consequence of vitiated air and other forcible adjuvants;—the pestilential vapours which arose from the soil were borne by the winds to the ships riding at a distance, and there fever failed not to manifest itself with its usual severity.

The actual amount of mortality produced by pestilential effluvia from the soil has never been accurately calculated in those countries where they are most severe. No bills of mortality or registers of deaths are kept, as in this country, in connection at least with the natives. But enough is known to shew that the amount is prodigious.

Tables are kept of the deaths occurring among the soldiers belonging to this country, serving on foreign stations, and they amply shew that the mortality is frightfully greater in those countries infested with these effluvia, and with the diseases which these effluvia are wont to excite, than at home—and as they are the chief agency of an unwholesome character, known to prevail in these regions, it is not unfair to attribute to them, in a general manner at least, a very great proportion of the excessive mortality.

The following extract, from an official return, will shew the greater mortality among the military when serving in the British Colonies than when stationed at home—

Official return of the mortality among officers and soldiers in the several British Colonies, chiefly for the seven years from 1820 to 1826, shewing the annual deaths out of ten thousand men.

Great Britain (1824 and 1826), out of 10,000 there died per annum,	144
Mauritius,	240
Madras Civil Service in 1820,	600
Ceylon, soldiers on the island,	1328
West Indies,	701

Such is the fearful mortality which occurs among our soldiers stationed in some of our colonies, where effluvia of a pestilential character exhale from the ground. In Ceylon, where terrestrial effluvia are known to prevail, the number of deaths of our soldiers is more than nine times that which occurs among those who are stationed in Great Britain.

The immediate cause of that frightful mortality is the malignant fever, the chief agent in whose production, again, is the pestilential atmosphere, rendered such by terrestrial effluvia, and not by the presence of specific contagious poisons, as defined earlier, assisted, perhaps, by other hurtful influences, such as, the intemperate habits which new comers in those colonies frequently adopt, the great heat of the climates, operating with particular force upon those accustomed to the more temperate climate of England.

This pestilential fever, the product of effluvia from the soil, commits such mortality among our gallant soldiery, as throws into insignificance the carnage attendant on active warfare, as renders that, even in the field of battle, comparatively of little moment.

Men in action may fall fast around; whole lines, nay columns of living humanity, its boldest samples, in one brief moment may be hewn down; still, as such carnage can last but a few hours of the day only, or, if protracted, a few days at most, the work of death is inconsiderable, compared with that effected by pestilential effluvia in many situations, operating both night and day, from day to day, and from year to year, unceasingly.

CHAPTER VIII

General Diseased Condition of the Body, the Product of Malaria

The inhabitants of countries infested with malaria, or vitiated air, when they have been spared the more acute forms of disease, or have recovered from them, are generally the victims of a miserable state of health, compared with which many conceive that death itself would be preferable.

The body loses its vigour and aptitude for exertion, becomes weak, disabled, sluggish, and impotent; the appetite fails: the limbs refuse to carry their burden aptly so called, and they become swollen and dropsical. The mind becomes lethargic and unfit for exertion, and the unhappy sufferer, who is insensible to whatever gratifies his more highly favoured fellow-men, becomes often weary of existence, a burden to himself, and an object of pity to others, who are accustomed to regard the activity, the cheerfulness, and graceful lineaments of health.

Thousands are so afflicted; and the number of those who thus have their existence embittered,—who are deprived of the manifold enjoyments which our condition can afford, and whose lives are prematurely terminated,—is even greater than that of those who die of the more violent and more speedily mortal distempers which are induced by vitiated air.

"A glance at the inhabitants of malarious countries or districts, must convince even the most superficial observer, that the range of disorders produced by the poison of malaria is very extensive. The jaundiced complexion, the tumid belly, the stunted growth, the stupid countenance, the shortened life, attest that habitual exposure to malaria, saps the energy of every bodily and mental function, and drags its victim to an early grave. A moment's reflection must shew us, that ague and fever, two of the most prominent features of the malarious influence, are as a drop of water in the ocean, when compared with the other less obtrusive, but more dangerous, maladies that silently but effectually disorganize the vital structures of the human fabric, under the operation of this deleterious and invisible poison."[7]

Such is the general state of health of the inhabitants of many parts of the world; but it is chiefly in some parts of "fair Italy," whose celebrated blue skies invite, whose luxuriant vegetation delights, whose gay and extensive prospects ravish, and whose classic associations charm the ecstatic spectator,—where humanity acquires that degenerate character, and that hideous aspect, which it assumes as if on purpose to mark the contrast between the gay revelry of vegetation, and the revolting degeneracy of mortality.

The resident in Italy can scarcely escape entirely the action of malaria; if he survive or escape the more immediate and more violent effects, those just described are, in the course of time, almost sure to manifest themselves.

Many of our countrymen make their residence in Italy, invited by its sky, its sun, its fertility, its ancient monuments, and stirring associations, and they not unfrequently prolong their stay so much as to imbibe the seeds of general bad health, which, though it may not develope itself at the time, will manifest itself at some future day. The malaria of Italy, like that of some other countries, sometimes acts slowly, and does not produce its effects, until the sufferer is again resident in his native country. Assailed with general decay, he is at a loss to know its cause, happening, too, at a time, when he had expected that his general health would have been more than ever established by his residence in a warmer climate, and under a clearer sky. It is a remarkable feature in the general bad health thus produced, that it is marked with periodical alternations of activity and repose, or with aggravations and remissions.

CRETINISM.

Cretinism, by which is meant a degenerate state of body, and an imbecile state of mind, which occurs for the most part in the valleys of Switzerland, and among the hollows of the

[7] Johnson's Diary of a Philosopher.

Alps and the Pyrenees, and that is in a great measure the product of vitiated air, emanating from the swampy valleys and basins, which contain animal and vegetable materials, powerfully acted upon by the direct and reflected rays of a burning sun.

From the mountains there pour many streams into the valleys or troughs beneath, and, as the water is seldom completely carried off, it there forms an excellent or very favourable nidus for the putrefaction of animal and vegetable remains.

It is said, by those who have attentively observed the miserable population in these regions, that they form the most humiliating picture of humanity. The body presents the most loathsome condition, and the mind is removed only a step from idiocy itself.

The unwholesome tendency of these terrestrial vapours is materially increased by the almost incredible filth in which the inhabitants keep their persons, clothes, houses, and streets, the effluvia of which alone are almost intolerable and most offensive.

The general degeneracy of the body is frequently accompanied with a large swelling at the front of the neck, which gets the name of "Goitre," and which is known in England under the appellation of "Derbyshire Neck."

Cretinism has prevailed in Switzerland for many centuries, and has been likewise noticed among the mountains of China.

Cretinism is thus ably described by Dr James Johnson: "The stature is seldom more than from four to five feet, often much less;—the head is deformed in shape, and too large in proportion to the body;—the skin is yellow, cadaverous, or of a mahogany colour, wrinkled, sometimes of an unearthly pallor, with unsightly eruptions;—the flesh is soft and flabby;—the tongue is large, and often hanging out of the mouth;—the eyes red, prominent, watery, and frequently squinting;—the countenance void of all expression, except that of idiotism or lasciviousness;—the nose flat;—the mouth large, gaping, slavering;—the lower jaw elongated;—the belly pendulous;—the limbs crooked, short, and so distorted as to present anything but a waddling progression;—the external senses often imperfect, and the Cretin deaf and dumb;—the *tout en semble* of this hideous abortion of nature presenting the traits of premature old age. The Cretins are voracious, and addicted to low propensities. To eat and sleep form their chief pleasures. Hence we see them, between meals, basking in nonchalance on the sunny sides of the houses, insensible to every stimulus that agitates their more intelligent fellow-creatures."

Before closing this sketch of the effects of malaria in Italy, a table of the annual decrement of life is submitted, which will shew the fearful mortality of that country over that of England, the disproportion against the former country being owing, in a very great degree, to the contamination of the atmosphere, caused by the effluvia which arise from the soil.

In Rome, 1 out of every 25 persons dies annually, or a 25th part of the whole population.

In Naples, 1 out of every 28 persons dies annually, or a 28th part of the whole population.

In England, 1 out of every 60 persons dies annually, or a 60th part of the whole population.

Thus, in England, the mean term of life is more than double what it is in Rome or Naples; and thus, while it takes 60 years to extinguish a generation in England, the brief period of 25 years completes the same work at Rome.

INTERMITTENT FEVER, OR AGUE.

Intermittent fever, more familiarly known as ague, is also a common product of air which is vitiated with effluvia arising from the soil.

That disease was much more prevalent some years ago in England than it is at present, where it is almost confined to Lincolnshire, and some of the low grounds and meadows of Kent and Essex, through which the Thames flows.

It is unnecessary to mention the symptoms of ague, as they are familiarly known. Convalescents are very liable to relapses, and many of those who have recovered from the more violent symptoms, are frequently affected, throughout the whole term of life, with very troublesome complaints, which arise from what is vulgarly known as ague cake, which is an enlargement of the spleen, an organ which lies near the stomach.

Ague is very prevalent in the West Indies, America, Holland, and other countries which are much covered with wood, are ill drained, and liable to be periodically inundated. This disease displays none of the virulence of the malignant remittent fever already noticed, yet affects vast numbers in its peculiar localities, and not unfrequently leads to mortal results.

The whole population of those fens and swamps in which ague is endemic, is generally affected at some period of existence, scarcely one person escaping.

The effluvia which produce that disease are sometimes carried to a considerable distance, and there induce their peculiar distemper; and instances are well known, where effluvia have been conveyed to high grounds, where they have attacked the inhabitants, while those in the immediate neighbourhood of the source of these vapours, have escaped for the time.

Ague is a much milder disease than the remittent fever, which springs from the same general source, viz. terrestrial effluvia, and which prevails in the East and West Indies, and on the coast of Africa.

When and where intermittent fever only is produced, it would appear that the effluvia from the soil are less virulent and concentrated, and perhaps their activity is modified or tempered by a proportionately great quantity of watery vapour combined with them in the atmosphere, by the climate of the country, and by the constitution of the people.

In this country, even so lately as half a century ago, ague or intermittent fever prevailed to a considerable extent, but is now almost unknown.

In East Lothian many of the old inhabitants remember ague as being a common disease in that county. At present it is there unknown.

In respect to this disease particularly, the health of the population of England has greatly improved, and it is well ascertained that the gratifying fact is chiefly owing to the country having been cleared of its superabundant wood, which prevented the land being readily dried, and which interfered with the due action of the winds, and to the speedy removal of water from the surface of the earth by draining, which is now so universally adopted. By draining, the water which formerly formed a receptacle for the decomposition of animal and vegetable remains, is now carried off, and with it the opportunity it afforded for the extrication of unwholesome vapours.

CHAPTER IX

Other Cases of Pestilence—Famine—Unwholesome Food and Drink

The operation of vitiated air in the production of disease is often very much assisted by the presence of other prejudicial influences.

It has been frequently remarked that one stroke of misfortune seldom comes alone, and that observation holds with striking force in reference to the causes of disease. One cause of disease produces another, which in its turn generates another, and so on, till the tendencies to, and the excitants of, pestilence, are so strong and so numerous, that whole communities are affected, one after another.

It not unfrequently happens that the predisposing source of some of the most severe visitations of the most virulent distempers, is the want of food, which generally depends on the exorbitant prices of provisions, raised either by the arbitrary regulations of rulers, or by comparative scarcity.

The total or almost total want of food is calculated to bring about, very shortly, a mortal result, from exhaustion or from sinking of the powers of the system.

When food is not withheld altogether, but is only given in sparing quantity, in an amount insufficient for the maintenance of the body in vigour, a condition of the system is induced, in which the functions are imperfectly performed, in which the blood and the various humours become universally prone to morbid change, and in which there arises a great tendency to disease of a low or asthenic character.

If, under such privation, vitiated air be present, whether arising from men in health, but uncleanly or crowded in close apartments; from the clothes, or excretions of the sick; or from terrestrial effluvia; it will give form to disease, will act as a spark amid fuel, and will shortly convert any predisposition to sickness that may exist into reality itself.

In those suffering under scarcity of food, there is generally experienced great depression of mind, which is hurtful in itself and injurious by preventing sufficient exertions for the maintenance of cleanliness: there is an inability to procure requisites for the purpose, and when, perchance, they are obtained, there is too often too much apathy or supineness to admit of their being used.

That miserable individual who is famishing, who is so unfortunate as to hear his helpless children call for bread, which he, alas, cannot give, who himself is exhausted and sinking with want, is seldom found to be very solicitous about cleanliness.

A mother so situated will, in her misery, amid her actual sufferings, and with the dark yet immediate prospect of further hardships, forget the necessity or disregard its call; of removing impurities from her hut, of retaining the persons and clothes of her family clean—and of washing the furniture, the walls and floor of her pestilence-haunted cabin.

In such a situation, cleanliness is neglected and impurities of all kinds accumulate which emit effluvia, to add to the number of the causes of gradual death impending over a family thus situated.

Let a case be supposed in which disease makes its appearance in obedience to the summons of so many forces, and let the malady be of a low or putrid character, and the patient dangerously ill. This family is unable from depression of mind, and from that exhaustion attendant upon actual want, to give him the requisite attention and assistance, and neither the means of cure are administered, nor is a suitable diet afforded. Effluvia arise, and no means being adopted to remove them, they become highly concentrated, and prove the immediate exciting cause of disease among all around who may be prepared by the operation of other favouring influences for that consummation. The occurrence of typhus fever among the labouring classes of this country, which is observed every winter, but more especially on those occasions when provisions, the necessaries of life, are high in price, when employment is with difficulty obtained, and when the wages are low, sufficiently attests the fact that scanty food is a powerful cause of disease, and one of a widely extended range of action. It is invariably in those years when there is least correspondence between the severity or inclemency of the season, the price of provisions and the means of the labourer that typhus fever commits most havoc. I have had occasion to note the prevalence of an unusual amount of disease, and amongst other forms, that of fever, in winters following partial failures of the crops, and the most satisfactory evidence has been afforded that a large proportion of the sickness was the consequence of high prices, and consequent scanty and insufficient food.

Such great prevalence of disease can be readily accounted for, when it is known that the ordinary amount of the wage of the day labourer does not exceed nine or ten shillings per week. I have heard labourers of the most sober and frugal habits affirm, that if their whole wage were spent in the purchase of oat meal for porridge, and of bread, that there would not be more of those provisions than would barely satisfy their children and themselves.

A scanty and unwholesome diet induces a bad and acrimonious state of the fluids, and leads to many diseases, and among others, to scurvy, which was long a frightful pestilence among our sailors.

Where there exists that tendency to scrophula, which is common in this climate, the relaxing influence of a poor and scanty diet is particularly hurtful, and proves the exciting cause of that hideous disease in all its frightful forms. Scrophula is much connected with a sluggish state of certain organs called glands. These organs are found in all parts of the body, and in health vary in size from that of a pin's head to that of a bean, but in scrophulous subjects they are found much larger, the smaller being often more than the size of a pea, and the larger being equal to a hen's egg.

Glands are congeries of vessels in which fluids of various kinds are elaborated, and it is partly from these fluids or those from which they are formed, stagnating in their vessels, owing to want of vital action, that the swelling arises, which is always found in scrofulous subjects.

That sluggish disposition of these parts is generally connected with a languid and lax state of the general system, which is liable to be greatly increased by whatever diminishes the vigour of the body. Few circumstances are better calculated to produce that effect than insufficient food, and hence it is that those diseases whose foundation is a scrophulous taint, are so much promoted in times of scarcity, and among individuals accustomed to a liberal diet when accidentally placed on scanty fare.

Instances are known where persons have become affected with weak eyes, with tenderness, watering and disposition to ulceration in these organs, immediately upon being put on spare and poor diet, and where a liberal supply of nutritious food has proved an almost immediate cure. That affection of the eyes was a form of scrophula, and fortunate it was for them that the form in which that disease manifested itself was not more dangerous. They had much reason to be thankful that the injury was capable of cure, and was not irremediable, as it has been in many instances, where the first intimation of the bad consequences of a scanty and insufficient diet has been decided and incurable consumption of the lungs.

When the glands which assume the scrofulous action are those of the lungs, and when they become the seat of the formation of matter, pulmonary consumption is said to be produced, a disease which annually carries off a great proportion of the adult population of this country.

Consumption of the lungs, or pulmonary consumption, is a common affection among those who subsist on scanty and insufficient food, and is frequently observed with dogs and other animals whose sustenance is small and precarious. Scrophula manifests itself in other forms, not less severe and extremely loathsome—in running sores on the neck and other parts, in swellings of the joints, and in various wasting diseases of the bones and their coverings.

In the various forms which this disease assumes, the blood and the different humours of the body become unhealthy and often acrimonious. The milk of nurses who are tainted with that habit is unwholesome, and when they are made to subsist on scanty and insufficient diet, it becomes poor, less nutritious, and positively injurious—and instead of being bland and white, it often appears watery and yellowish, and is irritating and acrimonious.

Food of an unwholesome or vitiated quality is also injurious, and has on many occasions proved to be the cause of much disease. Plants as well as animals are subject to disease, and food when obtained from such sources is highly unwholesome and detrimental to health.

The flesh of animals which have laboured under disease, has, on many occasions, done much harm, and is liable to be much more injurious than flesh which is merely putrid from being too long kept. Flesh merely putrid much more seldom proves hurtful, as, long before it can be very pernicious, it becomes so offensive that it cannot be consumed. Moreover, food which has acquired a slight taint, is more easily digested, its fibres become less tense, less hard, and more easily divided and dissolved in the stomach.

But the most important injuries of the kind have arisen from the use of diseased grain. On the Continent the rye sometimes becomes diseased, and the grain throws out a fungus somewhat like the spur of a cock. Rye thus deteriorated, when used for food, has produced disease of a very serious character. Persons who partake of it suffer great pain of stomach, fiery heat in the extremities, and very violent convulsions. This spurred rye produces mortification of the extremities, of a very remarkable nature.

The late celebrated surgeon, Mr Pott, thus describes these affections. "At the extremity of one or more of the small toes, in more or less time, it passes on to the foot or ankle, and sometimes to a part of the leg, and in spite of all the aid of physic and surgery, most commonly destroys the patient. It is very unlike to the mortification from inflammation, or to that from external cold. In its severer attacks, however, the constitution seems to be generally contaminated, the mind and body become equally debilitated, there is great irritability and a tendency to convulsive action."

Rye thus diseased produces another distemper, which partakes of the nature of typhus fever and that of plague: it is called by the French "Mal des ardens," and is generally considered one of the worst forms of the pest. That disease is marked by the most virulent character, and has, on many occasions, committed the most fearful ravages. It commences with a sensation of burning, prostration of strength, delirium, and vehement headach; a bad form of erysipelas attacks the skin, ending in suppuration, matter forms in the armpits and groins, and these symptoms almost invariably terminate in death. There is good reason to believe that the fungus or cock-spur is the product of disease in the plant. It is about the size of a cock-spur, is coffee-coloured, and may be readily detected when the farmer is disposed to use his eyes.

In this country, wheat which has been blighted or infected with the parasitic plant called mildew; has sometimes produced very bad effects, not unlike the severe burning at stomach, and the mortification which supervene on the use of spurred rye on the Continent. Not long ago, several families living in England were nearly destroyed by their using some diseased grain, which a farmer, knowing it to be bad, had sold at a reduced price. Other plants are sometimes known to be attacked with disease, and in that state are ascertained to inflict much mischief. The potato is more particularly injurious when its quality is bad.

Plants, like animals, may be affected with disease, and may be most unwholesome, without exhibiting any very marked signs of their morbid condition.

DRINK.

Drink is as essential as food itself, to the maintenance of the health of man. Thirst is no less urgent than hunger itself, and it often happens that it must be satisfied when the calls of the appetite for food are unheard. Drink of a wholesome quality is highly salubrious, and conduces much to maintain the blood, and the various humours in a healthy condition. Water is the only beverage with which Providence has directly supplied his creatures, and is, under ordinary circumstances, the liquid of all others the best adapted to their use.

Pure water is refreshing, cooling, and dilutes the blood, which, without some diluent, would become too thick to move readily along its containing vessels, to perform aright its manifold duties, and to accomplish its numerous purposes in the animal economy. Water taken into the stomach goes to supply that very considerable part of the mass of blood which is constantly earned off in the shape of sensible and insensible perspiration, and of other secretions, and to correct the tendency in that vital fluid, to become irritating and acrimonious from the formation and accumulation of various salts.

In order that the deleterious action of some liquids may be the more readily understood, we will inquire how drink, which is taken into the stomach, is there disposed of.

One of the chief objects which is obtained from the use of drink, is the dilution and mollifying of the blood; and in order that this important purpose may be effected, it is necessary that they be brought in contact and mixed with each other.

Water, or any watery beverage, being received into the stomach, many thousand vessels open their mouths upon the walls of that organ, and imbibe the contained liquid, in virtue of a vital action which they possess. The liquid is soon sucked up, and is carried by the veins and the absorbent vessels into the general circulation, there to be mixed and incorporated with the mass of blood. It has been popularly thought, that there exists a direct communication between the stomach and the kidneys, by which the contents of the former are conveyed to the latter organs; and that supposition probably arose from the fact, that the kidneys have an immediate increase of duty after copious drinking; and that fluids having a peculiar and strong odour have been detected, discharged, very soon after their reception into the stomach.

However, there is no direct communication between these organs, and all liquids which are taken into the stomach must be passed through the general circulation before they can reach the kidneys; and thus it is worthy to be observed, that liquids which are possessed of deleterious properties, have an ample field for their operation.

It is rare that any bad effects follow the use of moderately cold water in a state of purity, and any instances in which injury has followed, may, with perfect propriety, be regarded as depending on accidental circumstances.

It sometimes happens, that water free of impurities, cannot be obtained, and that, what is highly impure is taken into the stomach. Many nations are occasionally subject to the privation of pure water, and are compelled to have recourse to the tainted waters of sluggish rivers, of almost stagnant rivulets, and putrefying lakes; and the consequence is, that their health suffers, and that the invasion of disease is much promoted.

The inhabitants of Switzerland, and of several other countries, are supplied on some occasions, with no other water than that which is obtained from snow, and the prevalence of goitre among the Swiss, has been attributed by some physicians to that circumstance.

But man is not satisfied with this excellent beverage—water—which is ever at hand, and to be obtained without a price.

While yet little advanced in the knowledge of the arts, man discovered that the various juices with which the various fruits of the earth abound, afforded, during fermentation, a liquor which possessed properties such as strongly recommended it to his use. These juices, after fermentation, prove exhilarating and intoxicating, and all the nations of the world have their respective wines or intoxicating beverages. This liquor, which is the product of fermentation, gives to these juices their peculiar character. It is called spirits of wine, is colourless, and is lighter than water.

The liquors in which that active agent resides, when taken in small quantities, quicken the circulation of the blood, render more acute the perceptions, and augment the heat of the body. When these liquors are taken more copiously, the circulation becomes violently affected, the face flushes, and the blood is sent to the head, with too great velocity, and in too great abundance.

At first the mind is stimulated, but there gradually ensue sleep, stupor, and privation of sense and motion, which may continue even unto death. Several cases, in which death took place in this way from drinking to excess, are detailed in Mr Watson's excellent work on homicide. But when the quantity which is taken is insufficient to produce the last-mentioned effects, but is often repeated, it frequently happens that disease, more or less acute, attacks some of the more important organs of the body, as the stomach, liver, kidneys, brain, heart, and the general nervous system.

The diseases which follow the long continued excessive use of liquors, containing spirits of wine, vary in their nature, but, on the whole, they prove highly dangerous, interfere with the performance of some of the most important functions, and often lead directly to a mortal result.

Where death is not the immediate consequence of the diseased condition of these organs, symptoms arise which make the course of life run bitterly along, the general system breaks up, the miserable victim presents in vivid colours, the signs of premature decay, the accession of acute and mortal sickness is greatly favoured, and the intellectual faculties are impaired.

Many melancholy instances are known of soldiers at the sacking of conquered towns, who, indulging in wine and other spirituous liquors to great excess, have died in vast numbers, both immediately, and more slowly, through the operation of disease, which had been induced by too deep potations, by too long protracted carousing, and by that exposure to those influences favourable to the developement of disease, to which excess never fails to lead.

"Some thousands of soldiers covered the great square and the adjoining streets (of Moscow), but they lay extended and stiff in front of the magazines of brandy which they had broken open, and from which they had drawn death, expecting to derive from them life."[8]

The habit of indulging to excess in spirituous liquors, when it does not directly induce pestilence, assuredly lays those who are its victims, particularly open to its invasion, and is, therefore, entitled to be regarded as a very important agent in the great tragedy of life which is enacting.

[8] Segur's Expedition to Russia.

CHAPTER X

Causes of Pestilence Continued—Cold, Want of Clothing, and Shelter—Depression of Mind—Influence of Weather, Climate, Habits, &c.

Few of the primary causes of pestilence among large bodies of men are so powerful or so extended in the range of their action, as extreme and long continued cold, want of sufficient clothing and shelter, and depression of the mind.

Coincident with many of the epidemics which are wont to prevail in this country, these circumstances are almost, without exception, found to be present; and if they are not admitted to be considered as the sole and exclusive causes of the prevalent disease, it is proved that they are co-agents or adjuvants of the very first importance.

Much of the continued fever which infests the poorer classes of our countrymen, and almost all the pleurisies, colds, and consequent consumptions, which prevail more or less among the various ranks every winter, are in a very great degree dependent on the extreme cold of the season which suddenly sets in, and against which the dress of the inhabitants of these islands is insufficient to provide. The labouring classes suffer much, more particularly from the action of cold and the inclemency of the weather. They are generally very scantily clothed, nay, they are sometimes scarcely covered, and the consequence is, that the cold makes a strong and lasting impression, the circulation on the surface is suddenly impeded, the perspiration is checked, and the whole fabric involuntarily shivers. Now these are the very first symptoms of fever, and unless the constitution is possessed of stamina to remove those symptoms without loss of time, and to establish the circulation in its vigour again upon the surface of the body, that disease, or some other, will undoubtedly be established.

When a body thus affected with cold is placed in a warm

situation, there supervenes an excitement or reaction, which is marked by increased force of the circulation, and with redness and heat of the skin, a condition which is often experienced by persons who go immediately to the fire when newly arrived from a journey in the cold. When that reaction ceases, and is followed by a sense of coldness and by shivering, which again is succeeded by reaction, fever, in its proper sense, is established, and will assume a character of violence, lowness, or malignity, according to circumstances.

The clothes, the house, and the diet of the working man, are insufficient to protect him against the action of the cold, and to resist its operation when once it has fastened upon him; and thus it is, that to comparative want and to many privations, there is so often conjoined so much disease.

But it is in vain to expect any other result as long as our most deserving labouring population is worked in an inordinate degree,—so long as they labour beyond what their limited energies will, with impunity, permit—so long as they are often unable to obtain a diet sufficient for the maintenance, even of an idle person, and so long as their very breasts, from very want of clothing, are literally open and exposed to the fiercest blast that blows, and to the most searching and chilling rain that falls from Heaven.

Observe the industrious labourer at his work; behold his powers are taxed to the utmost, his energies, his capabilities, are put upon the stretch, and the entire fabric, God's most complicated and most delicate creation, is actually labouring and heaving with protracted exertion. His blood distils the dew of labour, and his clothes, such as they are, are moistened with perspiration bursting from a thousand pores.

It frequently happens, that the labour of the poor man being over, sorely fatigued, too exhausted even to enjoy the consciousness that his hour of rest has arrived, with a heavy and unwieldy gait and hanging head, he seeks his comfortless abode, his scanty board, his dreary, dark, scarcely furnished apartment, with its faint and glimmering embers.

He swallows his spare repast and falls asleep at his fireside, but having no change of clothes, and those which he has on being wet with perspiration or with rain, are allowed to dry upon him. In the mean time the heat of the fire proves sufficient to create a steam on the side next it, and the house of course being open to the wind, currents of air, chillingly cold, pervade the apartment, and strike upon that side of the poor inmate which is most remote from the fire, and thus he of a thousand misfortunes and privations is actually steamed on one side, and perished with cold on the other. Persons placed in such a situation can scarcely, for any length of time, escape disease, and it is consonant with my knowledge to say, that the condition of a great proportion of the labouring classes is not one tittle better. Fever and many other diseases will continue to assail our labouring population as long as their food is insufficient, as long as they are barely covered during the inclement season, and as long as their habitations scarcely own a roof or a door, as long as the wind and rain enter at a thousand crevices; and while the cheerful and salubrious light of heaven is denied admittance by the old hats, bunches of straw, and rubbish which so frequently, in the absence of glass, fill up the space originally intended for a window. Yes, so long as every energy is exerted, and every moment that can be cheated from rest, to obtain that wherewith a supply of the necessaries of life may be procured, and when every other consideration sinks and gives way to the more pressing wants of nature, will disease prevail.

Such is the destitution among many of the labouring class, and the vast amount of disease which prevails among them, is the necessary consequence.

The following facts illustrate well the influence which scanty food, insufficient clothing, and the privations attendant upon poverty, exert in the production of disease.

During the last three months (10th February 1839), the fishermen and potters living in Prestonpans, have been in a very destitute condition, the former, partly from the very boisterous weather which has prevented their going regularly to sea, and the latter from the closure of the potteries at which they were employed. During that time, these two classes of people have been suffering much from fever, about ten of their number having died in that short period; while the people, amounting to 750, including children, connected with Prestongrange colliery, who are well employed, well paid, and well fed, though inhabiting the same locality, and the houses stretching from Prestonpans to Musselburgh Links, have been almost entirely free of that disease, fever having affected two of those families only, in the course of the same time; and while fever is still prevailing extensively among the potters and fishermen, the people connected with the colliery have been entirely free of that disease since about the 7th of last December. On these facts I am well informed, being the medical attendant of the colliery.

Let us mark the operation of the same or similar circumstances upon soldiers; the consequences of exposure to cold, to the inclemency of the weather, of the want of sufficient clothing, and of habitations, among young and robust men, employed in the most active and spirit stirring occupations, connected with the most kindling and heart-rousing anticipations, and flushed with the glory and honour of victory.

Let the case be that of Napoleon's Grand Army in Russia, perhaps the most remarkable recorded in human history, and that, perhaps, will equal any that will yet mark the future career of man, in the total discomfiture, in the unspeakable sufferings, in the awful destruction of human life, and, in short, in the triumph of nature over humanity, which, from beginning to end, attended the disastrous retreat of that mighty congregation of France's bravest sons.

Let the case be that of the retreat of the Grand Army from Moscow, which, alas, was one horrid series of unprecedented disasters, of wreck upon wreck, whose course was one prolonged deathbed—one white, one snow-white shroud—one extended grave, which barely spared enough to convey the fatal tidings, and which received heroes by thousands, valour and all that is ennobling in the mass, which monuments can never note,—and broken hearts and broken ties, those of husband, of father, and of comrade, for which tears have flowed, but which tears can never bind again.

"At every step he (the Emperor) saw his soldiers, stricken by cold, extenuated by hunger and fatigue, falling half dead into the hands of the Russian cavalry.

"Around these (their bivouacs) hunger and cold rivetted those wretched sufferers. It was impossible to tear them away.

"Above sixty thousand men well clothed, well fed, and completely armed, attacked eighteen thousand half naked, ill armed, famished men, encumbered by more than fifty thousand stragglers, sick and wounded. For two days the cold and misery were so intense that the old guard lost a third, and the young guard one-half of their effective men.

"It was indeed but the shade of an army, but it was the shade of a grand army. It felt itself conquered by nature alone.

"Under these circumstances, the elements appeared more hostile to us than the Russians themselves. Their climate did its part—if they had done theirs."

In that disastrous retreat there was a most extraordinary accumulation of influences powerfully destructive of health. There was extreme cold, that of an intensely cold climate, there was an insufficiency of food and of clothing, and there was a want of proper habitations,—the wretched sufferers lying almost naked around their fires in the open air, perhaps enjoying the partial protection of a shed, a ruin, or a stable, and sometimes seeking shelter in the carcasses of horses. But there was also present another influence, highly prejudicial to health, and equal of itself to a considerable proportion of the fearful amount of disease which prevailed, and that was depression of mind.

Depression of mind conveyed a withering influence to the hearts of the bold victors of a thousand actions, and paralyzed the whole energies of the system. Here it acted on a gigantic scale, and its work of death, yes, of death itself, was not less prodigious.

The humiliation, the mortifications, and the heart-rending misfortunes of which these once victorious but now unhappy men were the prey, could not but induce a state of mind, which, of all other circumstances, must have been the most favourable to the invasion of disease. Daily experience demonstrates that disease is much favoured by the presence of circumstances, such as are referred to in the following passages.

"That grand army, which, in the course of the preceding twenty years, had marched in triumph through all the capitals of Europe, now, for the first time, reappeared, mutilated, disarmed, and fugitive in one of those (Konigsberg) which its glory had reduced to the greatest abasement. Its inhabitants hastened into the streets, as we passed along, to observe and reckon our wounds, and to estimate by the number and the extent of our misfortunes, the foundation on which they might build their hopes: we were forced to regale their eager and delightful eyes with our miseries; to submit to pass under the yoke of their delight, and, dragging our squalid and miserable forms in full review before their detested scrutiny, to march under the almost insupportable weight of calamity which the hatred of the spectators beheld even with transport."[9]

The very knowledge and observation of mental distress and bodily suffering creates a depression of mind, and sickness arising therefrom spreads among the spectators, although, in other respects, they are comfortably situated, and have abundance of clothing and wholesome food.

Segur further relates:—"Consternation took possession of the soldiers of Marshal Victor, though unbroken in numbers and in spirits, after having given way to their customary acclamations on beholding their Imperial commander, when, instead of the grand column which was to achieve the conquest of Moscow, they perceived behind Napoleon, only a band of spectres, covered with rags, women's pelisses, bits of carpet, or with dirty cloaks scorched and burnt by the fire of the bivouacs, and with feet wrapped in the most wretched tatters."

Depression of mind favours the accession of many diseases. This was noticed when the prevalence of fever was under observation.

It has been remarked by Citois, that the colic of Devonshire and Poutou attacks more particularly those families who are suffering under that calamity.

Disease frequently makes its first appearance when friends and relatives assemble to pay the last marks of respect at the funeral of the departed. I am acquainted with several instances in which, shivering, tremors, and sense of great debility, have suddenly supervened in men in perfect health upon the "lifting" of the corpse, and upon the "lowering" into

[9] Segur's Expedition to Russia.

the grave, moments in which the hearts of many would seem to threaten to melt away, and in which they have proved to be the primary symptoms of fever; the other more violent and more dangerous characteristics being duly developed. A man, named Stevenson, died at Tranent last winter; the friends were assembled in the house to attend the funeral; his brother arrived from a distance, just as the body was about to be lifted, went into the apartment, apprehended he smelt infection, and instantly felt very ill. After having gone to the churchyard, and returned home, he was immediately attacked with sickness, which assumed the form of fever, and he died in the course of a few days.

The following statement, made by Dr Paris, illustrates well, how depression of mind, by affecting the system, promotes the action of poison:—

"A patient had been taking mercurial medicine, and using frictions for a considerable period, without any apparent effect; under these circumstances, he was abruptly told that he would fall a victim to his disease; the unhappy man experienced an unusual shock at this opinion, and in a few hours became violently salivated (that is, became affected with the peculiar action of mercury on the mouth)."

CLIMATE.

Besides the various causes of pestilence to which reference has been made, there are many others connected with peculiarities of climate, irrigation, soil, and habitudes of nations, of which the limits of this work will not permit an extended account. Of the peculiarities of climate, the most important are the greater or less intensity of the sun's rays. It is found that much solar heat disposes to excessive action of the liver, and hence it is that fever in tropical regions is biliary; characterized by derangement of the biliary organs, of which the liver is the principal; that fever in the West Indies is yellow, a colour which proceeds from the dissemination of the bile throughout the body. Few persons who have remained long within the tropics are free of disease of the liver, and this is well known to be a common, nay, almost a universal complaint among soldiers who have returned to this country after many years' service in those regions.

Another active agent in the production of disease in these climates is the great fall of dew which takes place between the setting and rising of the sun, and the extreme degree of cold which attends it. The dew begins to fall as soon as the sun gets below the horizon, and increases till about an hour or two before dawn; the cold at that time is extreme, more particularly felt on account of the great heat which is experienced during the day. The cold is the immediate cause of the falling of the dew, which is only the water that was dissipated in vapour by the action of the sun's rays. The dew favours the action of the cold; and persons who are exposed to it, are in consequence frequently attacked with disease.

Persons unaccustomed to the heat, and ignorant or regardless of the consequences of exposure to the night air, often suffer much, and become affected with the peculiar distempers of the climate, in this manner: they lie down on the ground scantily covered, while the sun is still above the horizon, and make no provision for the cold and damp of night which is sure to overtake them.

Persons go to bed also with too few clothes, being then warm and oppressed with heat; in the night the dew falls, the cold arrives, and they are often awakened with severe rigors or shiverings; and thus fever, dysentery, and the like disorders are induced.

The winds in all latitudes are often instrumental in the production of disease. Some have been already referred to in connexion with the conveyance of vitiated air. Some are hurtful from their excessive heat, as, for instance, those blowing directly off the burning deserts of Arabia and of Africa. The Sirocco is not only extremely hot, but is copiously loaded with aqueous vapour. It visits Italy, blowing there several days at a time, and acts almost as a vapour bath upon the inhabitants. The Sirocco blows off the deserts of Africa, passing over the Mediterranean sea, there imbibing a large quantity of water, converted into vapour, and rushes upon the fair shores and degenerate population of Italy. Its immediate effect is to relax the system, and to open up all the pores on the surface of the body. These effects are very hurtful to health, and become particularly so, when they are long continued, as sometimes happens. But more dreadful are the results of exposure of persons so situated, to the sudden action of an intensely cold blast, such as the Tramontane, which, driving from the northern side of the Alps and Pyrenees, passing over their snow-capt summits, and sharing their bitterness and frost, rushes, without warning, upon the inhabitants.

The tramontane is very cold, and acting upon persons in a manner "forcing" in a hot house, soon produces pleurisies, colds, consumptions, &c. &c.

These vicissitudes in Italy, and those which are wont to occur in regions within the tropics, are much greater than the variations of weather which are experienced in the British Isles, and which are comparatively harmless; or are hurtful, at least, in a much less degree.

In many countries the rivers periodically overflow their banks and cover the surrounding territory. The Nile overflows annually, and when the water has almost disappeared by infiltration into the soil, and by evaporation, and when that which is left is muddy, slimy, and mixed with organized remains, exhalations arise, and a vitiated atmosphere is produced, which is said by medical men, who have lived upon the banks of that river, to be productive of plague.

The territory again on the banks of the Canton river in China, is almost constantly under water, and its fertility is thereby much increased. The ground there is used for the growth of rice which delights in a soil covered with water. When the heat is intense, when the water contains organized putrefying materials, and when the weather is close, and the atmosphere is a little agitated, then vapours ascend which, mixing with the air, cause it to be vitiated, and to be productive of malignant remittent fever.

The habits of nations are also influential in the production of disease. The privations and penances which devotees endure are followed by a very hurtful influence on the health, whether they be what are enjoined, or whether they be voluntarily suffered, as they suppose, to conciliate the favour of the Deity.

The diet, clothing, occupations, pleasures, government, laws, social usages, genius, and ambition of nations, materially influence their health, and give tendencies to particular maladies; but interesting as the subject is, the investigation cannot be pursued here.

CHAPTER XI

The Avoidance of Diseases Marked with Palpable Contagious Poisons—the Limited Range of Action of Contagion

It was shewn in the first part of this work, that the contagious poisons of disease, such as the matter of small-pox, are known to act in two modes only, *first*, by application of the palpable matter itself to a person, or by contactual contagion; *secondly*, by application of clothes or other such substances, impregnated with that matter, forming what has been styled fomitic or mediate contagion. It was also shewn, that their action through the medium of the atmosphere, has never been ascertained. Experiments were detailed, which were performed on those poisons, to ascertain their capability to become dissolved in the air, and their evidence was as strong as it possibly could be, against their possessing that attribute.

It was, in short, fully ascertained, that contagious diseases do not propagate by atmospheric contagion.

Contagious diseases propagate among those who expose their persons to contact with the matters or clothes impregnated with them. There are many facts of an incontrovertible character, which prove the occasional operation of the former mode at least, and to render probable, that of the latter; and hence, whatever attention is paid to cleanliness of the sick person, his apartment, and to the prevention and removal of vitiated air, persons touching a body, when there is present on its surface specific contagious poison, such as the matter of small-pox, or even handling clothes, which have become impregnated with it, incur a risk of being affected with the same disease, by means of that matter or fomitic contagion.

In all the contagious diseases (those in which there is eliminated a palpable poison, or matter capable of causing the same disease in others), their respective matters are invariably formed, and are apt to propagate in the modes specified, so that visitors and other attendants should ever be upon their guard, the first not to touch the sick person at all, and the latter not to touch more than is necessary, and to take precaution to render the risk as slight as possible.

Subjoined is a list of diseases which are known to be contagious, or to be possessed of a matter of the nature referred to, and that are therefore wont to be propagated by contact with the sick, or with his clothes.

Small-Pox.
Scarlet Fever.
Measles.
Chicken-Pox.
Cow-Pox.
Itch.
Plague.
Porrigo.
&c.

These are almost the only diseases known in this country, which are positively ascertained to be characterized by the elimination of contagious matter, and which, therefore, there is any risk of getting by contagion. The continued fever of this country has been supposed, by some physicians, to be a contagious disease, from there being sometimes observed pimples on persons affected with it; but that is by no means an ascertained point.

Those above enumerated seem to include all the most important diseases in this country, which are capable of being propagated by contagion, acting in either of the two ways already described. Some of them are capable of affecting the same individual only once, and some affect persons as often as they are exposed to their specific contagious matters.

How comparatively small, then, is the range of contagion,—an agent which has been thought to accomplish worlds of mischief, and to destroy almost whole communities.

Visitors may approach within a very short distance of persons afflicted with these distempers, without danger of suffering, provided they do not touch the bodies or the clothes.

They have nothing to apprehend from the atmosphere, if attention is paid to the maintenance of its purity,—such as is necessary in other situations, as well as in the sick-room.

Never brought into that immediate contact with the poisons which is necessary for their propagation, they stand in need of no directions for their removal or counteraction.

Those persons, on the other hand, who are called upon to touch the patient and his clothes, are exposed to danger; and they should lessen its amount, by instantly putting their hands into warm water, and by freely washing them, with the assistance of soap,—and that ablution should be performed after each instance of contact.

I have often had occasion to feel the pulse of persons ill of the worst forms of confluent and black small-pox, and any risk that has thereby been incurred, has been removed or remedied by immediately washing the hand as directed.

In addition to washing, after that process is done, a small quantity of a strong smelling liquid, such as Lavender water or Eau de Cologne, should be poured into the hands. Their grateful odour may hide or cover that of the apartment, which the attendant may mistake for contagious air, as is often done, and thereby remove groundless apprehension. These seem to be the chief precautions that are necessary for meeting the dangers of contagion, if there is included what is sometimes used, viz. a covering for the hand,—a glove and the like,—which, as being harmless, and such as may possibly be useful, should be employed; and likewise the avoiding of eating and drinking with the same instruments and vessels used by the sick persons.

The propagation of disease by contagion, in the modes already stated, though it can take place, and though it sometimes does take place, still there are the strongest grounds for supposing it a comparatively rare occurrence.

I have already shewn, at the beginning of this work, that in one form, the atmospheric, contagion never operates, and I am now prepared to assert, that in the two forms in which alone it can act, that the instances of its undoubted agency are by no means nearly so common as they are commonly believed to be, especially in connexion with those acute diseases, accompanied with fever.

It is my belief, founded on much observation, study, and reflection, that almost all cases of those contagious diseases, arise from causes or circumstances connected with those great agencies already detailed at full length, as inductive of pestilence in general, and of a nature epidemic, endemial, meteorological, and the like.

I am led to the opinion, that this course of origin, even in contagious diseases, is the rule, and that the origin of disease, by contagion, whether contactual or mediate, is the exception. The grounds of this opinion are,—

1st, A fact well ascertained, and of which I had lately two instances, in houses contiguous. Infants neither inoculated, nor vaccinated, lie with their mothers and others ill of small-pox, and do not take that distemper.

2d, Women, while labouring under small-pox, occasionally bear children in perfect health.

The above are common occurrences, and I am in possession of the particulars of several which came under my own observation in the beginning of 1838.

These cases prove the occasional, nay, the frequent inactivity of contagious poison, even when applied in a palpable form, and in a recent condition, to the bodies even of those who are not protected against its operation by inoculation for cow or small-pox, or by a previous attack of disease; and this inactivity is observed too, when the most ample opportunity is afforded for the action of the poison, viz. while children are asleep together in the same bed, and when infants are upon the breast of mothers affected with small-pox.

Those very children who thus escape taking disease by contagion, are frequently known to be seized with that identical disease, at some future time, varying from months to years, when no other case is known to exist in the neighbourhood, and where there is no room to suspect the operation of contagion.

It is, I believe, as common as the contrary course, for small-pox, and other reputed contagious diseases, after appearing in one house in a town or hamlet, to break out in others at a distance and in different directions, and not to progress from that which was first attacked to those lying adjacent, or to spread around as from a centre.

For example, the first case of Typhus Fever which occurred in my practice, in January 1839, was at Meadow Mill, a village half a mile north of Tranent; the second case was at a hamlet called Redcoll, about four miles east; the fourth and fifth cases occurred in Tranent; while the sixth and last for that month appeared at Elphinstone, a village situated about two miles to the south-west of Tranent.

I am led also to the opinion, that the ordinary cases, even of those diseases which are known to be occasionally propagated by contagious poison, do not arise from contagion, but from other circumstances and agencies; by the history of the plague, for while that scourge is ravaging in the East, and destroying hundreds daily, it frequently ceases, immediately upon the overflowing of the Nile, which buries and covers the pestiferous soil, and the putrefying materials which had been exhaling noxious emanations.

This sudden departure or cessation of plague, upon the overflowing of the Nile, proves that contagion, though it may be the cause of some cases of that disease, is not the occasion of the vast majority,—the great mass of cases, in short, which constitute the Epidemic; and goes far to prove that distemper to be dependent upon an unwholesome condition of the soil, or vitiated atmosphere, and other widely extended and unwholesome agencies, of a nature totally different from specific contagious poison.

That fact goes to prove, in reference to one disease, viz. Plague, what I believe holds with all other contagious distempers, that contagion, at most, is only an occasional, while such influences as those to which reference has been made, are the constant and general causes of sickness.

CHAPTER XII

The Prevention and Correction of Vitiated Air

The important part which vitiated air enacts in the production of many forms of disease, has been already fully shewn; and it must be admitted, that whatever has for its objects the prevention and correction of that principle, is deserving of attention.

By preventing the production, and by removing vitiated air when already formed, a vast amount of disease may be arrested, and much of that benefit will actually be accomplished, which it was boldly but fallaciously pronounced would revert from many absurd measures which were adopted, and which are still recommended for the avoidance of contagion, and would realize almost all the advantages which Quarantine Regulations, and the most efficient systems of Contagion Police can or propose to afford; and that, too, at no inconvenience to individuals, no restraint upon communication, after certain processes of purification have been undergone, and no ruinous hindrance of commercial transactions.

The various sources of vitiated air have been already noted. Some of them are beyond any present remedy, as the unwholesome condition of the surface of the earth in many regions, within the tropics, for whose correction or improvement, time, capital, enterprise, labour, and perhaps new climates, are essential. To that source of vitiated air, draining, cutting down superabundant wood, embanking rivers, reclaiming partially inundated land, and cultivation, must be applied before the emanations which infest these situations can be prevented from arising.

Another source of vitiated air is, men being crowded together in close and confined apartments, where no attention is paid to the preservation of cleanliness and the removal of impurities, as in some jails and other places for the confinement of criminals.

That source of vitiated air is particularly worthy of notice here, because a very common form of disease which it induces is what is well known as Jail or Contagious Fever.

The means for the prevention of this form of vitiated air are obvious. Large, airy, well ventilated and lofty apartments are essential, if many persons must be put together; and, where that is not necessary, it is advisable to have them separated in several different chambers, where due ventilation is strictly maintained, by retaining the windows more or less open through the day, or by other equally effective means.

By the sleeping of many persons in one apartment, the atmosphere is deprived to a great extent of its more vital fluid, and becomes unfit to support respiration in its integrity; and the health of the inmates is not unfrequently injured in consequence. The sleeping of many persons in one bed-room, therefore, should be avoided, where it is possible; but, where that is not practicable, it becomes necessary to lessen the evil consequences, and this may be done by keeping a door or window partially open during the night, when the weather is not too inclement to forbid that procedure.

At all times, exhalations to a great extent are proceeding from the bodies of men; and, where individuals are much confined to one apartment, and where that is small, close, and ill ventilated, they fasten or adhere to the furniture, curtains, carpets, and the very walls. During sleep, the amount of these exhalations, it would appear, is increased. It is then that the pores of the entire system, as well upon the internal as the external surfaces, are most freely laid open, and that they pour forth their respective fluids most abundantly. The quantity of watery vapour which issues during sleep from the lungs is prodigious; and the large quantity of water which is sometimes seen collected on the panes of windows in the morning, and which is condensed vapour, affords some idea of the vast quantity of fluid which is exhaled during sleep. With this watery vapour, other ingredients of a hurtful nature are conjoined, and, like it, adhere to the furniture and clothes. When these exhalations are permitted to remain, they impart to the room a disagreeable odour, cause the bed-clothes to be damp and unwholesome, which, with the progress of fermentation, at length emit offensive effluvia. In order to avoid these hurtful consequences, the following measures should be adopted. When the bed-room is left in the morning, the window or windows should be opened, and the bed-clothes freely exposed to the air for some time: the constant passing of fresh air over the clothes and through the apartment, will shortly carry off the greater part of the exhalations which may have adhered.

The window should be left open during a part of the day, if the atmosphere without is not particularly damp, as the removal of impurities, when they have adhered to solid bodies, is not effected at once, or so immediately as is generally believed.

Exhalations of a very hurtful nature proceed also from excretions, which should be removed immediately, certainly before fermentation can have proceeded to any considerable length.

The furniture of bed-rooms requires special care. The various processes of rubbing, washing, and scouring, should be frequently repeated; and articles, such as bed and window curtains, should be oftener in the washing-tub than is dreamt of by many very careful housekeepers, and when they are composed of fabrics of a nature to forbid contact with soap and water, the necessary purification may be effected, at least in a partial manner, by occasional exposure to the wind in the open air.

In those apartments in which the sick are contained, the atmosphere is particularly liable to become vitiated from the exhalations of the body, and from the excretions being in general more disposed to be virulent than those of persons in health.

The necessity for a constant supply of pure air is, if possible, increased, and the utmost care and attention is demanded, in order that this may be duly provided. In large hospitals for the reception of sick, ventilation becomes a point of the most important nature; and, when efficiently established, is entitled to be considered one of the most powerful remedies which can be obtained to check the progress of disease, and to promote recovery, when that is once established.

Various methods have been devised to promote ventilation in hospitals, which it is unnecessary to describe here; for this reason, as well as others, that the importance of ventilation is too well understood by medical men, for them not to enforce it in establishments of which they have the management.

During sickness in private houses, ventilation cannot be too much enforced. When the weather will permit, one window at least should be partially opened, pulled down, if possible, during the summer. In winter, the door of the apartment should be left open for a short time occasionally; and, if the chamber is not very small, a fire may be used, which will not only remove the cutting dullness of the air, but will also ensure a constant change of the atmosphere, from the ventilation which it causes.

In some forms of disease, as in the "Sweating Sickness of England,"—the typhus fever, the skin is wont to become covered with perspiration, which is particularly prone to undergo putrefaction. To obviate that putrefaction, and to prevent the formation of effluvia, it is proper to wash the skin of the patient, in almost every form of disease, with soap and warm water, which will purify that important organ, and assist in rectifying its functions. Where the character of the disease is putrid, sponging the skin with vinegar and water, either warm or cold, should be adopted, and is often of the greatest use.

All impurities should be removed from the sick-room, as they are liable to vitiate the atmosphere; and all clothes and utensils which have been used by the patient should be immediately put among warm water, and left there till a convenient season occur for their being thoroughly cleansed.

When the patient is in a state to bear the fatigue of being removed for part of the day to another chamber, advantage should be taken of his absence from his bed-room, to ventilate the apartment, by throwing open the doors and windows, to expose his bed and body clothes to the free action of the air, and to cover the sickly smell frequently present in sick chambers, by the burning or dissemination of some fragrant substance in the atmosphere.

CORRECTION OF VITIATED AIR.

The effluvia which are wont to arise in sick-rooms, are sometimes so very strong, especially where little attention is paid to cleanliness and ventilation, as to fasten most tenaciously to the contents of the apartments, and to impart to them a most disagreeable and sickly odour, not immediately removeable upon the establishment of currents of air obtained by opening the doors and windows.

These effluvia, for the most part, are cognizable to the organ of smell, and they have long been, and are still, vaguely designated "Contagion," "Infection," and the like.

Where effluvia are not recognised by the organ of smell, there are many good reasons for believing, notwithstanding that circumstance, that they may be present in rooms which contain, and which have lately contained, sick persons.

Well authenticated cases are on record, where persons in health have inhabited apartments which, at a former period, contained sick persons, and have been attacked with disease in such a manner as to leave little doubt of the presence of unwholesome effluvia, and of their having been the efficient agency in the production of the evil. These instances have occurred, where it is impossible to suppose that the effluvia could have been commingled with the atmosphere during the whole interval, often amounting to years, from the period of the removal of the sick, to that of the taking up of their abode there by those who have suffered.

The period during which the apartment has been uninhabited has, on many occasions, been too long to admit of the opinion that the atmosphere has not been again and again changed. It would therefore appear, that not only the atmosphere becomes infested, on those occasions, with effluvia, but that the walls, the furniture, and the floors may likewise become impregnated with them.

It is consonant with experience to admit, that solid bodies occasionally combine with, or imbibe, or attract gasiform products, or that aeriform or vaporic agents adhere to solid substances.

The opinion may be entertained, that the effluvia of sick

rooms may fasten to the furniture, &c., and in that situation, even where ventilation is maintained, form centres from whence they may be disengaged, either constantly, for a long period, or only on occasions which are particularly favourable for their redissemination in the atmosphere.

It is common to designate these effluvia primarily disseminated in the atmosphere, and the vitiated air which is formed in old fever and plague wards, and to which reference has just been made, Contagion, without any other term to mark the distinction between these principles and those which are legitimately so called. In a previous part of this work, the distinction has been carefully made, and it was shewn that the effluvia under discussion do not form, strictly speaking, a contagious, but only a vitiated atmosphere.

As it appears that effluvia which arise from the bodies, and the excretions of the sick, do not only mingle with the atmosphere, but also adhere to furniture, walls, &c., when concentrated and long exhaled, it becomes necessary not only to remove that atmosphere in which they are disseminated, but also to adopt means for the purification of all those bodies to which they may adhere, in order that the atmosphere may not become again and again loaded with them, arising, as they may, from the places to which they are adhering.

The means best calculated to obtain that end, are those processes to which reference was made above, viz. rubbing, scouring, washing, and exposing to the free action of the air.

But besides these means of purification, there are others, as fumigations, which are calculated to be highly useful, and which should be used on all occasions of severe general disease.

Fumigations are vapours of an elastic nature, permanent and non-permanent. They are diffused through the atmosphere, and impart to it their peculiar odours.

They are highly useful. In the *first* place, there is reason to believe that they, especially the more active, may decompose the effluvia which are mingled with the atmosphere, and which are adhering to solid bodies, all of which they can be made to reach and act upon, and even to penetrate where the scrubbing-brush and hot water cannot be applied; in the *second* place, they insure a change of atmosphere; and, in the *third* place, they effectually cover or hide the smell of the sick-room, which is at all times highly disagreeable, and which is often regarded with great terror and apprehension, being ever associated with ideas of contagion and disease;—and in this way, fumigations are found of very great value, giving, at the same time confidence to the timid, and affording something different from what contagion is commonly thought to be, on which the organ of smell may be safely exercised.

Some fumigations are produced by the volatilization of solid bodies, as camphor and carbonate of ammonia, or sal volatile;—some by the volatilization of liquids, such as vinegar, pyroligneous acid, and the various essential oils, as cinnamon, rose, thyme, mint, pennyroyal, carraway, and turpentine, while others are permanently elastic fluids or gases, as muriatic acid gas, chlorine, and ammonia.

The first-mentioned substances, viz. camphor and ammonia, are not very strong, and may be disseminated through the apartment of the patient, even when he is present, without giving him any uneasiness. Carried about with those who visit the sick, and who are apprehensive of contagion, they are useful by affording a grateful odour, which hides disagreeable taints, and perhaps it is in that way chiefly that they are useful.

The liquids which have been named above, have been long used for the purposes of fumigation, and in general, they may be employed even in the presence of the patient. A few of them may possibly decompose effluvia, but there is much reason to think that they are useful, for the most part, by hiding ungrateful odours, and imparting to the atmosphere, which is liable to be suspected as unwholesome, a delightful fragrance.

Vinegar is much used for the purpose, and with very considerable benefit, and is therefore to be employed.

The essential oils are capable of being diffused throughout the air, and with the assistance of heat, are often made available for the purpose of covering odours. When they are to be used, the oils should be poured upon a piece of live coal, held in the middle of the apartment; they are then immediately converted into vapour. In like manner, vinegar and the other volatile liquids may be disseminated through the atmosphere.

The oils, the vegetable substances in which they are contained, tar and the like, are occasionally burnt with the same intention, and sometimes with advantage.

The incense so much used by the ancients, was procured for the most part by the burning of the vegetable substances in which these essential and fragrant oils resided, by which part of them is diffused in vapour.

The ostensible and pretended object of the priests, in offering up incense, while that and other religious rites were performing over the bodies of deceased persons, was the conciliation and propitiation of the Deity. But while this was the sole ostensible object of the priests, and that which was held by the people, as the only and exclusive purpose proposed, there is good reason to believe that the offering up of incense, like many other observances of religion, had its temporal, and worldly, as well as spiritual ends; and that the sweet smelling odours, which were thought would be so grateful to Heaven, were, on those occasions, used in no small degree, as so many fumigations, to defend the pious and resigned priests from the effluvia of the dead body, and the consequent corruption of the atmosphere.

The use of fumigations, in a disguised form, was perhaps rendered necessary, as the purpose of purifying the atmosphere, might have seemed to cast reflections or imputations on the dead, which the vile, barbarous, and superstitious people, especially relatives, might have resented with acts of violence, or which might have thrown priest-craft into contempt and abhorrence.

Perhaps it was in reference to this matter, as it was in many others of graver import, that the ignorant and superstitious condition of the people on the one hand, and the cunning, subtlety, despotism, and superior knowledge of the ministers of religion on the other, in early times, made it convenient that certain ends, thought to be desirable, should be accomplished without reasons, explanations, or intentions being given.

There is, then, reason to believe, that the burning of

oils and other fragrant substances, was used in very early times to purify the atmosphere from the effluvia of dead bodies.

The products of the combustion of essential oils, tar, pitch, and the like, are carbonic acid gas and watery vapour, which, there is reason to think, cannot be useful in purifying the air, or in neutralizing hurtful effluvia.

The permanently elastic gases which are used as fumigations, are the most potent agents of the kind, and they are generally used, and with much propriety and advantage, in all cases where disease is of a putrid character, and where, in short, the atmosphere is likely to be vitiated to a great extent. They form also the most useful fumigations for the purpose of purifying the atmosphere, and the walls and furniture of apartments lately inhabited by the sick, and their employment, in such cases, should never be neglected, even when there is no great reason to apprehend vitiation of the atmosphere, for when advantage is doubtful, there can exist no possibility of detriment. The agent now most commonly employed, is chlorine gas, and it is perhaps the most efficient in the list of fumigations.

Chlorine gas has a greenish colour, and a most disagreeable and suffocating odour. Water impregnated with it, has the property of destroying colours, and chlorine is, on that account, much employed in bleaching, in the forms of "Bleaching Powder" and "Tennant's Powder."

When chlorine gas is disseminated through an apartment, any stench, however strong and intolerable, which may have been present there, is no longer perceptible, the odour of the chlorine taking its place, or so completely covering it, as to render it no longer cognisable to the senses.

Chlorine gas is employed both alone, and in combination with other bodies, as lime and soda.

In combination with these alkalis, chlorine forms the chlorides of lime and soda. The former is well known in this country, and the latter, when dissolved in water, forms the "Liqueur disinfectante" of Monsieur Labarraque, which is much celebrated on the Continent.

The solutions of these salts in water, are sprinkled occasionally through the apartments which are to be purified.

When these solutions are sprinkled about, and exposed to the action of the air, the chlorine escapes in its gaseous form and mingles with the atmosphere, while the lime and soda, which are now uncombined, attract and unite with any carbonic acid which may have arisen from the patient, his clothes, or excretions.

The solution of chloride or chloruret of lime, answers sufficiently well, but as it is to be obtained in all drug shops, it is unnecessary to add here a formula for its preparation.

FORMULA FOR THE PREPARATION OF CHLORINE GAS.

Take three parts of common salt, one of black oxide of manganese, and three of strong oil of vitriol. Mix the salt and the oxide together in a stoppered retort, pour in the oil of vitriol and apply a gentle heat. The gas is immediately evolved, and rapidly diffuses itself throughout the atmosphere. Muriatic acid gas, a combination of chlorine and hydrogen gases, though considered as inferior to chlorine as a fumigation, is frequently employed for the purpose of decomposing effluvia, as the materials for its preparation are almost ever at hand.

FORMULA FOR OBTAINING MURIATIC ACID GAS.

Put a handful of common salt previously made very hot into a saucer, and pour over it an ounce of strong oil of vitriol. The gas is immediately extricated.

It has been already said that the fumigations just noticed are on many occasions highly useful, and their employment is much recommended in all situations where the atmosphere is liable to be contaminated by effluvia from sick persons or from dead bodies; but it is not therefore to be understood that, because the use of these agents has been advocated, it is for the purpose of destroying atmospheric contagion, of decomposing the specific animal poisons which have been supposed to be present, and dissolved in the atmosphere, which is the object, or one of the objects, held in view by the generality of those who advise the use of fumigations. These fumigations have been recommended with the view of correcting what has been treated of as vitiated air, which is distinct from, but which has long been erroneously regarded as, Atmospheric Contagion. On some occasions, great fires of wood, coal, pitch, gunpowder, and the like, have been recommended for the purpose of destroying contagion and purifying the atmosphere. During the prevalence of the plague in London, great fires were kindled in the streets, and, according to some historians, with considerable benefit.

Such great fires produce great agitation of the atmosphere, and it is possible that in this way they may prove useful in improving the condition of that fluid, particularly when, as happened occasionally during the visitations of plague in London, the weather is sultry and close, and when the atmosphere is confined and little agitated, and allowed almost to stagnate.

There is much reason to think that the agitation of the ocean, by its waves and tides, is not more favourable to the preservation of the purity of its waters, than the movement of the atmosphere, by winds and currents, is to the maintenance of its wholesome condition, and when this is lost, to restore it; and in the absence of winds, and when pestilence is raging, the use of combustion on a large scale may with advantage be adopted; but in this climate, where the weather is seldom long calm, the occasions for the employment of that agency can be very rare indeed.

Heat is much used for the purpose of dissipating effluvia, and purifying goods, clothes, letters, &c., which are supposed to be impregnated with contagious matter, or other unwholesome impurities; and there is good evidence to shew that this agent is perhaps the most powerful instrument which is ever employed for the purpose in question.

Heat when applied to an atmosphere containing effluvia will rarefy it, cause it to become lighter, and dissipate it, amid the atmosphere above, where any opportunity is afforded for its egress; and when the heat is employed in the sick chamber, much good is effected by the dissipation of the damp and condensed vapour which cannot fail to be frequently present in that situation.

In the sick chamber, the presence of a fire for even an hour daily is highly useful where there is little opportunity for ventilation, and when the external atmosphere is damp and motionless, for the heat issuing from it, will dislodge and dissipate any effluvia which may have become condensed, and have fastened on the furniture of the apartment.

The condensation of effluvia, &c., is thus depicted in the "Mussulman." The apartment is that of a prison. —— The pestiferous breath of the surviving was mingled with the effluvia from the dead, and the empoisoned exhalation was condensed on the damp walls, and was seen trickling down in drops of poison to the ground.[10]

Heat, when applied to clothes which are impregnated with specific contagious matter, or merely impurities or condensed effluvia, is calculated to be highly useful, and where washing cannot be adopted, should never be neglected. Clothes which are thus tainted will be deprived in a great measure of their power of doing mischief, by placing them before a fire for a considerable time, for there is good reason to think that specific contagious poisons will be decomposed, and it is ascertained that condensed effluvia may be dissipated by the application of a smart heat.

The following experiment will at once illustrate the property which some bodies possess of absorbing effluvia from the atmosphere, and prove the influence of heat in again expelling and dissipating them. Pure sand, exposed to a red heat to drive off impurities, was put amidst tainted air. Put into a glass tube and exposed to a spirit lamp, it yielded ammonia or hartshorn,—a product of putrefaction which the sand had undoubtedly absorbed from the tainted atmosphere. Ammonia is a compound of nitrogen and hydrogen, gases which are evolved during the putrefaction of animal materials.

The investigation of the means by which persons, merchandize, clothes, letters, &c., may be most speedily and most effectually freed from effluvia, contagion, and other unwholesome impurities, is a most important point, for it relates to the most vital interests of society, commerce, freedom of intercourse, personal liberty, and the safety and health of the community. But from the very important considerations with which the investigation is connected, the

[10] The Mussulman by Madden.

merits of the respective means employed for the purpose will not be treated of here, as they deserve a more extended consideration than can be given. In the mean time it would be highly dangerous and impolitic, to adopt any great and rash change in a system so important as quarantine, until the most full and sound inquiry has been made upon the subject. Public safety demands the utmost caution.

There may exist great diversity of opinion respecting the nature of the impurities with which merchandize and clothes are sometimes impregnated, on the period during which they retain their activity, and on the means of purification; but it has been often clearly demonstrated, that specific contagious matter, or virus, and effluvia, may be conveyed by these bodies, may be retained for a considerable time, and, on a favourable opportunity, produce very hurtful effects.

The impurities may be variously designated, yet their unwholesome tendency is much the same, and it is necessary to adopt provisions to counteract it.

CHAPTER XIII

The Prevention of Vitiated Air in Connection with the Disposal of the Dead—Offals—Construction of Towns, Houses, Sewers, &c.

In the Chapters which have been dedicated to the subject of Vitiated Air, its sources were pointed out in a general manner, and it is intended to consider those usages in society, certain conditions of towns and houses, and some other circumstances, which favour the production of an impure and unwholesome atmosphere, and this will be done with the hope that a knowledge of their hurtful tendency may lead to their correction.

The disposal of the dead will be first considered.

As soon as the life of man is extinct, his body becomes the seat of chemical decomposition or putrefaction, and effluvia are exhaled from the putrid corpse, varying in some degree, in amount, rapidity, and activity, according as the circumstances in which it is placed are more or less favourable to putrefaction.

The effluvia which are exhaled are deleterious, and an atmosphere in which they are evolved, if close, small, and confined, often becomes so contaminated and vitiated as to be calculated to produce death by suffocation and disease.

The body of man after death is thus a centre of putrefaction, and the source of agencies prejudicial to the living, and on that account alone, it is wise so to dispose of the dead that they may not prove hurtful to the surviving, which has been done with more or less efficiency from the very earliest epochs of time, by various forms of burial.

But solicitude for the safety of the living has not been the only motive for the burial of the dead, for the destiny of man after death is clearly pointed out, and his doom to the earth is amply shewn by various expressions contained in the Holy Writings, and his burial or interment has been performed in obedience to the original or divine plan.

The interment or burial of the dead has likewise been considered as a rite due to the memory of the deceased, and a mark of respect which the friends and relatives were bound by every sacred obligation, to perform with all becoming solemnity.

To neglect the sacred office of interment, or any of the solemnities usually in practice, was, even among the earliest Greeks and Romans, to treat the memory of the departed with the grossest disrespect and indignity.

The denial of burial, with all its formalities, was esteemed by the Greeks as a mark of infamy due only to villains, traitors to their country, and those who died in debt, and the bodies of such characters were accordingly decreed unfit for ordinary interment.

The Jews interred the bodies of the dead for the most part contiguous to the high ways, in gardens, and on hills.

The Greeks and Romans interred their dead in the ground which surrounded their sacred buildings, and at the gates and porticoes of their temples.

The Saxons, Danes, and other Scandinavian nations, enclosed the bodies of the deceased in stone coffins, which were placed or built at the distance of two or three feet from the surface of the earth.

At this day, these stone coffins are occasionally discovered at a little depth from the surface. Some such coffins were lately discovered in the parish of Gladsmuir, in East Lothian, by the coulter of the plough coming in contact with them. On examination, the coffins were found to be only a foot and a half below the earth's surface:—they were about five feet long, and were composed of several stones fitted together, or built up. Within were found human bones of the adult size, quite entire in figure, but so friable, as to fall to powder along with the clay in which they were imbedded, on being handled. The vertebræ or bones of the spine, which are at present in my possession, present the same accuracy of outline to be found in the recent skeleton.

The situation at which these coffins were found, is the very summit of Seton Hill, a point which commands a view of the surrounding country to a very great extent, and of the

Forth, from its mouth to its meanderings in Stirlingshire, and which there is much reason to think, may have been at a very early time, a Danish or Saxon encampment.

The Hindoos dispose of their dead or dying by throwing them into the Ganges, where they rot and decompose.

In this country the dead are interred at a much greater distance from the surface than was practised by the Scandinavian nations, generally at the depth of five, six, or eight feet, and sometimes even more.

After death, corpses are usually kept several days before interment, and as the temperature of this climate is seldom very great, bad effects are very seldom experienced, and in that respect, Britain is very unlike some tropical regions, where, almost as soon as death has taken place, it becomes necessary to bury the bodies of the deceased in order to avoid the noxious vapours, which are immediately emitted.

During the time the corpse is kept before interment, attention should be paid to secure a full and frequent change of air, which is best obtained by keeping the windows partly open, by volatilizing vinegar, or by sprinkling the apartment occasionally with the solution of chloride of lime.

The mode of burial of the present time, which is practised in this country, is, partly from accidental circumstances, a great improvement upon that which was in use by our ancestors; for there is much reason to think that effluvia, proceeding from dead bodies, may percolate or be strained through a covering of soil of only two or three feet, which may be completely confined by one of earth and stones of five or six feet in depth. The great depth to which graves are now dug, originated not so much with the view of preventing the percolation of effluvia, as with the intention of embarrassing the operations of the bodysnatcher, whose violation of tombs is now happily at an end. But though there now remains no occasion for adopting measures for that purpose, the good practice of deep burial to which that evil gave rise should not be allowed to go into desuetude from the absence of those circumstances which called it into existence.

It is agreeable to information which has been gathered from various sources, to state, that effluvia may and do penetrate through the loose soil and other materials of churchyards, when the body is placed within three feet of the surface of the earth.

With that covering, effluvia do not escape in large quantities at a time, so as to produce very serious and instantaneous effects; yet a small amount may percolate from time to time, which, by acting constantly, without intermission, may be the mean of deteriorating or undermining the health of those persons who live in their immediate neighbourhood, and more especially if the situation be one which is not readily accessible to winds and currents.

It is stated by grave-diggers, that when a body is interred in a grave five or six feet deep, the effluvia do not reach the surface; so that it is evident that deep graves are much less dangerous to the living, and should be adopted in preference to those which are shallow. It is much to be desired, that no more burying-grounds should be opened or formed in the heart of towns, and that those which are at present in use, in such situations, be entirely closed against the admission of more bodies, and that cemeteries be opened at some distance from the habitations of men.

Every good purpose which is at present obtained from the burial-grounds situated in towns, might be also procured from cemeteries placed at a little distance in the country; and many disadvantages might be avoided in the latter situation, which attend burial-grounds in densely populated situations.

One great advantage to be obtained from exurban cemeteries, is the freedom which the population would enjoy from those exhalations which must ever arise, in a greater or less degree, from overcrowded burial-grounds which have, for any considerable time, received the remains of the dead, and a consequent improved state of health.

Deep graves may for a time prove a security against effluvia, but a day must come when these graves will be opened, and when their contents, perhaps not yet totally assimilated with the surrounding clay,—not yet completely deanimalized,—will be thrown to the surface, and mingled with the soil, there to finish the process of decomposition, and there to vitiate the atmosphere.

The burial-grounds of our densely populated towns are actually supersaturated, if such an expression can be used, with the partially decomposed remains of mortality, which have not yet had time to be assimilated with the earth, or to be "ripe," as the grave-digger would say.

In general, also, those burial-grounds are so small and ill-proportioned to the wants of the population, that it is necessary to open graves, and heap body upon body, until they reach to within a very short distance of the surface, or to clear the ground of its contents while they are yet green, in order to procure a place of rest for other bodies.

Such is occasionally the scarcity of ground, small though that space be which will suffice for any one individual, that ere a few short years have rolled away, the intrusive spade of the indifferent sexton disturbs the grave, perhaps of a friend,—that place where peace was promised and through life expected;—his ashes are rudely handled, and his bones, not yet denuded of their flesh, are cast without remorse amidst the rubbish;—and thus the best feelings of humanity are outraged, and the human heart, already wrung with anguish, is crushed or cruelly lacerated.

It will perhaps be urged in reply, that the vicinity of burial-grounds in the large towns of Great Britain are not more unhealthy than other quarters.

But the answer to this is, that no extended and minute inquiry has been instituted on the subject; that though the absolute amount of disease may not be increased (which, however, has not been shewn), still, a part of the disease which does occur, may arise from the operation of the emanation from the burial-grounds; and, lastly, it must be obvious to all who are sensible of the advantage of a pure atmosphere, that the effluvia which necessarily prevail in those situations, must be prejudicial to health, whether it be in an amount, or intensity, or mode, to admit of the detection of the relation between them, as cause and effect.

If, perchance, in some instances, no prejudicial influence is exerted upon the health of persons inhabiting the neighbourhood of burial-grounds, that fortunate immunity from the ordinary effects of effluvia arising from decomposing animal remains, accumulated in large quantities, is to be attributed, not to the innocence or innocuous nature of the emanations, but to the wholesome influence of winds and currents, in securing a constant supply of pure air, and which prevent the accumulation of these gaseous poisons in quantities sufficient to produce the bad effects which are commonly experienced in situations where they are much concentrated. It is almost impossible to adopt measures which will completely prevent the admission of effluvia from burial-grounds into the atmosphere, and it were therefore wise that the evil, a necessary one as it would appear to be, should be made to exist where it is least likely to do harm,—and that situation is certainly in the country, in the open fields, where there are few or no houses.

It is to be hoped that the subject of exurban cemeteries will shortly obtain the consideration of the government of this country, and of the magistrates of the various towns,—as it involves interests of the most important nature.

Several large towns have already cemeteries at a little distance in the fields; and among others, Glasgow has its City of the Dead, or Necropolis, as it is styled, which is situated on a height adjoining the town.

Paris, the capital of that country which has produced many of the most eminent chemists, has not been tardy to avail itself of the light which their philosophers have thrown upon the composition of animal bodies, and the chemical constitution of the atmosphere. That capital boasts a magnificent cemetery, called Pere la Chaise, which is situated at a little distance in the open country.

Pere la Chaise is becoming, as the Place of Rest of the dead, worthy to hold the ashes of departed mortality. There the bodies of men can in no way be hurtful to the health of those who survive; there, now incapable of being useful, they are at least harmless to that community of which they lately formed a part. There the silence—the proper silence—of the tomb is maintained; there a serenity of aspect exists, which comports well with the solemn, the quiescent state of its inhabitants; and there is a cheerfulness, and a beauty, aye a brightness, of a softened, and a mellowed kind, which seem to refer to the pure enjoyments of the promised land. There, as in the burial-grounds situated in our thickly populated towns, there is no obvious and striking unwholesomeness, no offensive and humiliating appearance of mortal remains, to deter from a casual glance, or from entrance on the part of the friends and relatives of the departed. On the contrary, in Pere la Chaise, they are invited and allured by the softened and chastened beauty of the place, and there, without endangering their health from close and vitiated air, they linger by the ashes of the dead, and revolve those solemn thoughts, so wholesome and so heavenward bending to the soul;—there the bereft parent is seen giving the reins to his feelings, fondly recalling cherished associations, and there he is learning to hear unappalled that he must share a like fate with that of the object whose grave he now regards;—there may be seen the orphan, come to shed the tear of filial love over the manes of his departed parents, reviving ties and affections which are too liable to be entirely worn away by youthful enjoyment, and the various unsubstantial fascinations of the world;—and there he learns that most useful and wholesome lesson, to look with complacence, if not with prospective joy, on death and its silent abode,—to divest himself of that dread and horror often excited by these ideas, and which, alas, too frequently drive the young from such considerations altogether.

In Pere la Chaise, a murmur is heard proceeding from the town, and the impression made upon the mind is, that the world is receding, that the noise, mirth, and tumult of man is vanishing away, and that, in short, the reign of death has commenced,—the reign of death, solemn but not terrific.

How different is the abode of the dead in the bustling commercial towns of Britain. Here, solemnity is incongruously enough and offensively mixed up with the noise and bustle of every-day concerns of men bent on business or pleasure. Reflections on eternity are here interrupted, perhaps by the music, or rather the ungrateful noise, of a musical instrument being played in an adjoining street, the rolling of carriages, the trampling of horses, the smacking of whips, and the indecent oaths of waggoners;—while in another street, or fashionable promenade, which the eyes of the mournful visitor of the abode of death cannot possibly avoid, the ill comporting sight is seen, fine ladies and still finer gentlemen laughing and tittering, busied with fantastic displays. 'Tis an ill-assorted scene, 'tis Nature burlesqued beside humanity defunct.

But the improvement in burial-grounds is urged, not on the plea of feelings and sentiments, but on that of public utility and general health.

THE CLEANSING OF TOWNS.

Until within a comparatively short period, the large towns of this country were kept in a very unclean condition, from the accumulation of impurities; and the consequence was, that there prevailed a vitiated and most offensive atmosphere, which often proved hurtful to the health of the inhabitants.

Habits of cleanliness, and proper notions of domestic comfort have made rapid progress of late years, and fortunately all classes of the community enjoy clean and wholesome apartments and streets, compared with those occupied by their ancestors of a century back; and families at the present day, who belong to the middle class of society, have the advantage of greater cleanliness, both of house and locality, than was then enjoyed by persons of the higher classes.

In many large towns an admirable system of cleansing is maintained, by which the removal of impurities is insured, which might taint the atmosphere. The laudable endeavours of the magistrates for this purpose, have uniformly met that ready cooperation from the more respectable portion of the inhabitants which they so well merit; but with the lowest classes, whose ideas are too coarse to permit their recognising danger in such things as uncleanliness and impure air, the suggestions of philanthropic individuals, and the exertions of authority, have failed, in a great degree, to produce that wholesome condition of houses and localities which is so desirable.

Much uncleanliness still prevails in some streets in those quarters of towns occupied by the labouring population, which proves the source of many effluvia, which again, it is probable, assist much in the production of the great amount of disease which is wont to prevail in those parts.

There is reason to fear that a considerable proportion of the lowest classes in all large towns is too much degraded to give themselves any concern about lessening the tendencies to disease, or to put themselves to any trouble to remove impurities, further than is absolutely necessary for their own convenience; but, in such instances, the authority of the law should interfere, and compel compliance with regulations for that purpose, the infringement of which is calculated to produce consequences prejudicial to the public health.

Many, nay most, of the villages of Scotland are kept in a most offensive and unwholesome state of filthiness; large heaps of corrupting animal and vegetable materials being allowed to accumulate, in many instances, in the public thoroughfares, and before the very doors and windows of the houses, proving the source of the most abominable effluvia, offensive to the senses of those who are accustomed to a pure atmosphere, and injurious to the health of all who inhale them. Trenches or hollows are, in many instances, to be found before the doors, where water is collected, and forms a nidus for the putrefaction of the materials above mentioned, and whence issue effluvia which are often to be recognised in the houses.

In these hollows or cavities are thrown all sorts of impurities, and they are allowed to remain till a cart-load or two have accumulated, when, if sufficiently decomposed, they are sold as manure to farmers and others, at the rate of about a shilling the cart-load.

The collection of impurities is in this case not the result of apathy and laziness, as in the purlieus in large towns, but of the desire of gain, or of a trifling advantage, such, for instance, as getting a small piece of ground, rent free, for the growth of potatoes, which is a common practice.

Very bad consequences attend the unwholesome condition of the atmosphere always found in these situations, and more especially in warm and close weather.

The quarter of Tranent in which typhus fever prevails most is that called Dow's Bounds, and a more filthy part is not to be met with in Scotland; a large area in front of the houses being completely occupied with the cavities aforementioned, with their putrefying contents, and the place being ill adapted for ventilation, forming three sides of a square, and the ground having no declivity, nor efficient sewers to carry off the rain, the most favourable circumstances exist for putrefaction, and for the contamination of the atmosphere.

In the construction of future towns, and in additions to the old, the utmost attention should be given to promote the free agitation of the atmosphere, if it is proposed that they should be salubrious. Where health is to be protected, the streets should be made wide, open, and occasionally terminating in squares or other open places.

Where circumstances will permit a choice, towns should be built in wholesome situations and dry soils; and the same holds with additions making to old towns.

The health of a community is much influenced by the situation in which they live, and by the nature of the ground on which their houses are built.

In many towns there are some particular districts in which disease is more particularly prevalent, and the result of careful inquiry is, that the excessive disease is owing to unwholesomeness of situation. Persons in all other respects similarly situated, enjoy a better state of health, or suffer less disease, who inhabit a more wholesome or less prejudicial situation or locality.

SEWERS.

A point next in importance to a proper construction of streets, and the selection of good situations, is an efficient system of drains or sewers for the removal of impurities, and the formation of water-courses.

Of the importance of sewers it is unnecessary to enlarge, that being sufficiently understood.

By water-courses is meant channels for the immediate passage of rainwater from off the streets. They are easily formed, and where the ground is level, the advantage is very great. In streets having a slope or declivity, the water is soon dispersed; but where they are level, it is apt to collect, and there create dampness, which is communicated to the houses, and a favourable nidus for putrefaction, where impurities are permitted to accumulate.

In some parts, principally the suburbs of large towns, and in many of the villages of Scotland, perhaps more especially those along the coasts, inhabited by fishermen, no means being adopted to expedite the removal of rainwater, and there being no natural water-run or course, the rain collects, and animal and vegetable materials mixing therewith, green putrefying ditches are formed, plentifully evolving gaseous products, and supporting a luxuriant vegetation on their surface.

CONSTRUCTION OF HOUSES.

So much attention is now paid to health and comfort in the construction of the houses of the wealthy, that it is unnecessary to say a word respecting these points, in connection with the higher classes.

But the circumstances being so very different in relation to the houses of the poor or the labouring class, some notice is required here.

It too often happens that the house of the labouring man in the country is, in almost every respect, little better than a shed, and calculated to produce disease. The walls are frequently the only substantial part of the tenement, the roof of tiles being often pervious to the rain and wind, and there being no other covering either of lath or lime; the door opens directly into the body of the house, and the floor is generally either below or on a level with the ground outside.

When floors of houses are below the level of the ground outside, they must necessarily be damp, and cause the house to be unwholesome.

The floors even of cottages should be situated about a foot or more above the level of the adjacent ground, and the interval between them and the soil should be filled up with small stones, or such materials, and then the houses might possibly be free of damp, and the rain would not run in off the streets, and form ditches before the very fire-place, as it does in many houses in this village.

The necessity of the floors of their houses being at a little distance above the ground is well known to the natives of Manilla. To avoid the dampness and the unwholesome emanations of the soil, the poor natives build their bamboo houses upon a foundation of wooden piles, by which contrivance a considerable space is left to permit the winds to enter, and to dissipate the damp and exhalations. In like manner, the rich inhabitants of Manilla build on piles of brick. Could our working population, or rather their landlords, not take a hint from these less refined people, and form some security against that unwholesomeness inseparable from damp houses?

It is unnecessary to detail at length instances of the greater prevalence of disease among the inhabitants of low-lying, confined, damp, ill ventilated, and filthy towns, over the populace of cities more favourably situated in these respects.

It will suffice to say, that typhus fever prevails more in the Old Town, where there are many local causes of disease, than in the New Town of Edinburgh, where the streets are clean, wide, and well drained;—and that the plague prevails more in the Jews' quarter, remarkable for the filth and closeness of the streets, than in any other part of Constantinople.

CHAPTER XIV

Prevention of Disease by an Active and Cheerful State of Mind, Sufficient Clothing, and Wholesome Diet

The bad effects of despondency and apprehension have been already stated, and they were found to be very important and highly favourable to the invasion of disease. Instances have already been given of disease and general decline of health following depression of mind and long continued apprehension, and it now remains to point out the salutary action of an active and cheerful state of mind.

An active and cheerful state of mind imparts an activity to the various organs of the body, whereby their functions are more perfectly performed; it spreads a kindly glow over the entire system, and tends to dispel any sluggishness of action present in any part which perhaps would, under other circumstances, increase, and lead to the development of disease.

On some occasions a cheerful state of mind, induced by sudden improvement of prospects, or by the unexpected receipt of good intelligence, has been the efficient instrument in dispelling the first symptoms of disease which had been induced by depressing causes.

It has been often observed among soldiers and sailors, who, losing their health and beginning to suffer from disease, under no other apparent unwholesome cause than the distrust with which they regarded an insufficient and unskilful commander, that their health has suddenly improved, and disease has rapidly diminished when they have been put under an able chief in whom they reposed confidence, and with whom they were willing and ready to place the safety of their lives.

Soldiers and sailors suffering many privations, mortified with defeat, failing in their energies, and beginning to drop under the influence of disease, have, on the sudden and unexpected brightening of their prospects, regained their lost strength, cast out the seeds of disease, thrown off their despondency, and have achieved worlds of enterprise. The following interesting case, which illustrates well the powerful influence of hope, and a cheerful state of mind, is taken from Paris's Pharmacologia.

"In the celebrated siege of Breda in 1625 by Spinola, the garrison suffered extreme distress from the ravages of scurvy, and the Prince of Orange being unable to relieve the place, sent in, by a confidential messenger, a preparation which was directed to be added to a very large quantity of water, and to be given as a specific for the epidemic; the remedy was administered, and the garrison recovered its health; when it was afterwards acknowledged that the substance in question was no other than a little colouring matter."

That impaired state of health, and much of the disease, especially of the digestive organs, which is so much experienced by persons who are suddenly deprived of much occupation of the mind in business, and find themselves totally unemployed, and who, from their previous habits, are unable to derive enjoyment from literary and scientific pursuits, as some retired tradesmen, have been suddenly removed, and health has been fully re-established on the individuals being again immersed in business, either from choice or by a happy reverse in their circumstances rendering that step unavoidable.

During epidemics, that confident assurance which some persons are known to entertain, that they will escape the prevalent distempers, there is much reason to think, has on many occasions been a complete prophylactic or preventive.

Instances are not uncommon where an assurance or settled conviction on the part of the patient has gone far to promote, if not to produce, recovery from very dangerous disease, when physicians have despaired of life, and even when that opinion has been communicated to the unmoved and still confident sufferer.

The history of amulets or charms and of the cures performed by the royal touch, affords much amusing and interesting detail illustrative of confidence and hope, in the prevention and cure of disease. Instances are also familiar of naval and military officers who have lost their health from the long continued suffering of "hope deferred" in respect to promotion, and of neglect of meritorious services, where advancement and the grant of their longing and earnest wishes has at length acted as a charm upon every bodily ailment, and where a rapid succession of cheerfulness and health has been the immediate consequence, to the joy of anxious and apprehensive friends.

The beneficial effects of activity and cheerfulness of mind in warding off the attack of disease, and in promoting recovery therefrom, having been so strikingly illustrated in the above examples, there remains no occasion to say more than to recommend them strongly for adoption, both among those in health and in sickness.

CLOTHING.

The want of sufficient clothing as productive of disease has been already noticed.

Clothing in this climate is used for the purpose of retaining the body warm. Now this is an important purpose, and the means by which it is attained are highly deserving of notice, and they exert a very powerful influence upon health.

The temperature of the human body is generally about 98° Fahrenheit, and that of the surrounding atmosphere being in this climate always below, sometimes in severe winters, as for instance the last, being near zero.

Now, all bodies possess a property by which they are disposed to maintain an equilibrium of temperature, that is, to be of the same amount of heat, and the temperature of the human body being above that of the surrounding atmosphere, in an amount varying at different times, it parts with a portion of its heat, or caloric, as it is called by chemists, which is communicated to the atmosphere and surrounding bodies.

A portion of the heat of the body is constantly, and under all circumstances, being abstracted by the atmosphere and other surrounding bodies which are at a lower temperature, and were it not that the loss of heat, which the body is thus constantly sustaining, is supplied by the formation of heat in the system, which is ever going on, the body would soon become so very cold as to be incapable of performing its functions, and death would consequently ensue.

The amount of heat which the body loses, and the rapidity with which it is abstracted, is proportionate to the coldness of the atmosphere and surrounding bodies.

But the rapid and great abstraction of heat from the human body, which is apt to take place when it is immersed in a very cold atmosphere, is very hurtful, and often induces disease, especially fevers, colds, coughs, and inflammations.

It is for the purpose of checking the rapid abstraction of heat from the body, that the warm clothing used in these latitudes is adopted. It is a bad conductor of heat, and the consequence is, that the temperature of the body is not reduced so rapidly as it would be were it exposed without any covering to the atmosphere, which, more especially when damp, is a superior conductor of heat.

Clothing of a sufficient nature is useful in the preservation of health, by preserving in its integrity the circulation of the blood on the surface of the body, by maintaining the constant flow of the secretion from the skin, or perspiration as it is commonly called, which is so useful to the system in many different ways, and by preventing any deviation from that balance in the distribution of the fluids of the body which that process goes so far to maintain, much to the comfort and freedom from disease of the individual.

Many instances of a very striking nature are known, where such inveterate and mortal disease has supervened in consequence of the privation, total and partial, of clothing, and from that being of a texture and nature inadequate to meet the exigencies of the case. Some have been referred to in this work where the want of sufficient clothing has been one of many concurrent potent circumstances, the attendants and consequences of poverty and destitution which have given rise to epidemics. On occasions of great distress and destitution, the disease which is then so very prevalent is not the product of one circumstance merely, such as want of food, but is induced by the many concurrent powerful and unwholesome influences to which poverty is ever sure to give rise. One of the chief circumstances on which the wide prevalence of disease depends on those occasions, there can be little doubt, is insufficiency of clothing among the poorer classes. But it is the advantages which are to be derived from sufficient clothing which should here occupy attention. Of late years, it has been the practice in some towns in this country, on occasions of fever and other diseases prevailing during the cold and inclemency of winter, for funds to be collected for the purchase and distribution of clothes among the poor and ill-clad portion of the population.

The motives and feelings with which this form of charity has been adopted, must of themselves be a sufficient and highly delightful return for the liberality and exertions of its benevolent projectors and supporters, but it must afford them much gratification and much encouragement in their laudable and christian endeavours, to know that the clothing which they have dispensed has had a powerful influence in preserving many from becoming the victims of the prevalent distempers, and of preventing the relapse of the convalescent.

The late Sir John Pringle, a distinguished army surgeon, states that "the best clothed were generally among the most healthy regiments."

The quantity of clothing should of course vary with the season, more being used in winter than in summer. A minute account of the outer clothing is unnecessary here, but a word may not be thrown away; the body should at all times have that quantity of clothing which will secure it from unpleasant feelings of cold and chilliness, and it would be wise to be influenced more by comfort and a regard to health, and less by fashion and caprice in the choice of clothing, which is so intimately connected with the preservation of health and its unspeakable comforts and enjoyments.

The clothing which is next the skin is more important, and will here obtain some consideration. It may be laid down as a general rule that flannel or some such woollen cloth should be used next the skin throughout the entire year. It will be well to vary the cloth or flannel in different seasons, perhaps using a thick flannel during winter, and a material of lighter and less close texture during summer and autumn. A fabric of fine flannel, or what is called "stocking," answers very well for the summer, when the flannel which is commonly used is felt to be too warm and irritating to the skin. In the summer it is common for many persons who use flannel during winter to discontinue its use, but it is safer, merely to exchange the thick flannel which has been used during winter for one of a finer fabric or some such equally fine material.

During winter when the weather is always cold, and in spring when it is generally chilly, flannel or some such material should form an essential portion of the clothing of every inhabitant of these islands.

It is safe to say that hundreds in this country are at present alive and enjoy excellent health who, but for the use of flannel and such like fabrics next the skin, would have been, ere this, numbered with the dead; and it is not too much to say that thousands are at this moment in perfect health through the kindly action of the same clothing, whose lives were threatened with constant coughs, periodical colds, quinseys, rheumatisms, and incipient disease of lungs, and other organs of the chest, before this efficient guardian of health was adopted.

Flannel and fabrics of the same or like nature go far to preserve an equable temperature at the surface of the body, promote the perspiration of the skin, which they readily absorb when copiously secreted, and are specially useful in preserving the balance of the secretions on the surface and in the interior of the body. Now all these most important conditions, which the use of flannel goes so far to maintain, are ever liable to be subverted and disturbed, whenever the body is thinly or inadequately covered, by changes in the ever varying temperature of the atmosphere, and by the prevalence of winds and currents.

Most of the important constitutional diseases which occur in this country, begin with a sensation of coldness with shivering and trembling; now it is the usual property of flannel, and such fabrics, when worn next the skin, and indeed of warm and general good clothing, to obviate and prevent these conditions of the body, and thus disease may be met at its very onset, and perhaps baffled ere it has time to establish its dominion.

"In some situations my personal experience enables me to vouch for the utility of flannel. Of this we had a very striking proof in the second battalion of the Royals, while suffering from a most aggravated form of dysentery in India. General Conran, the late Lieutenant-Governor of Jamaica, who at that time commanded the Royals, was so fully persuaded of the benefits likely to accrue from the general use of flannel, that he went down from Wallajahabbad, where the regiment was then stationed, to Madras, on purpose to represent to the government the distress of his men, and to suggest the expediency of a supply of flannel shirts. This he did with so much effect, backed by the late Dr Anderson, the Physician-General, that the flannels were immediately ordered, and, in my opinion, contributed much to check the alarming progress of the disease."[11]

It is usual with many individuals to wear flannel only over the chest, but it is wise to envelope the whole body in that most useful article of clothing.

The poor or labouring man should endeavour to procure thick soled shoes, in good repair, and substantial worsted stockings.

The latter are generally esteemed stronger and more durable when made at home, and will form excellent work for his wife or daughter in the winter nights.

The working man will find, that though clothing substantially, as has been above recommended, takes a considerable proportion of his money immediately out of his pocket, he will be a certain gainer in the end, aye, probably in the course of a few years or months, by consequent immunity from disease, and from continued capacity for labour.

FOOD.

It has been already shewn in this work, that the want of sufficient and wholesome food is frequently attended and followed by disease. It is now proposed to shew how important food and drink, of good quality, are to the preservation of health; but the fact is so well known, and so undoubted, that it is almost unnecessary to say that they are essential to the preservation of the body in its strength and

[11] Ballingall's Military Surgery.

dimensions.

That sense of sinking and languor, which is so commonly experienced upon long fasting, would soon be exchanged for the actual pains of disease, were it not to be removed shortly by the taking of food.

When the body is exhausted from the want of food for some hours, a good and ample repast imparts strength to the body, and cheerfulness to the mind, and goes far to prevent the evasion of some forms of disease.

An individual who is well fed, is generally more secure against the invasion of disease of a low character, than another who is only scantily and occasionally supplied with food.

It is generally believed that individuals who have lately partaken of food, are less subject to the operation of vitiated air, or as it is commonly termed, "contagious air;" and it was commonly reported during the late prevalence of cholera, that persons who took breakfast before going out, suffered less from that disease than those who followed a contrary course.

Many well authenticated instances are recorded of the health of armies undergoing very great improvement, and of disease in these bodies being greatly checked by the distribution of ample wholesome food, and by the privation which they had suffered for some time previous, being ended, by some accidental circumstances, as the gaining the enemy's magazines, or the reduction of a siege. Sir George Ballingall relates in his work on Military Surgery, that "during the prevalence of a malignant fever in this regiment (33d), then stationed in the garrison of Hull, in the autumn of 1817, amongst other measures calculated to check the rapid extension of the disease, I recommended the regular supply of breakfast to the men. This was immediately ordered by the commanding officer, and nothing appeared either to the officers, to the soldiers, or to myself, to have so much effect in obviating attacks of the fever."

The institution of soup kitchens in this country, for the distribution of wholesome and nourishing food to the perishing poor, there is no doubt, has a most salutary influence in the prevention of disease, by, in short, so fortifying individuals, otherwise incapable of resistance, as to render them proof against the influence of many causes of pestilence.

There can be little doubt that the liberal distribution of nutritious food, which of late years has happily taken place from these charitable institutions, has gone far to check the ravages of fever, which is so prevalent in this climate, during winter, when the labouring classes are subject in so great a degree to cold, and the privation of food and other necessaries of life.

It is stated on good medical authority, that no measure which was instituted for the purpose of stopping the progress of typhus fever in Glasgow, in the winter of 1837–8, then very prevalent and mortal, was so useful, and so immediately and obviously efficient, as the establishment of soup kitchens in that city.

Among the arrangements in Edinburgh in 1832, which tended apparently to render cholera less extensive than in other large towns, a soup kitchen formed one.

Fever has been much less prevalent in Tranent during the present, than for many winters past, and this is to be attributed partly to a soup kitchen which has been instituted in that village, and which has been in operation for about two months (16th March 1839).

The excellent tendency of such establishments must be obvious to all who are at all conversant with the nature of disease, and the animal economy, and it can form no valid objection to that proposition, that fever is still known to have raged where soup kitchens have been established; for, though the pestilence may not have been extinguished, still it may have been abated, and though the malignant character and mortality may not have been reduced, still these excellent institutions may have been the means of preventing their being increased.

Let not, therefore, those who are willing and able to support whatever is calculated to reduce the sufferings and privations of the poor, be driven from extending their support to soup kitchens, because they have only diminished the number of the victims of disease, and made the stage of convalescence more sure and less liable to relapse.

It would indeed be vain to expect, that the distribution of

food would act as an entire preventive of fever and disease, which is the result not of scanty food only, but of that and many other circumstances of a very different nature, whose operation, the supply of soup, in any quantity, can go a very short way only, to remedy.

Some of the circumstances which exert the most important influence in the production of pestilential disease, and the measures which are best calculated to counteract their pestiferous tendencies, have now been detailed.

It is hoped the enforcement of the hurtful operation of many circumstances, erroneously thought to be innocent, may lead to their being remedied in future, and it is expected, that if the suggestions which have been thrown out in the latter part of this work, are duly acted upon, or if others of a like nature, which may, at a future period, emanate from another better qualified for the task, should meet with the attention, which this object so well demands, the amount of disease will be diminished, human suffering will be abated, and human life extended nearer to that point of maturity which the Divinity has decreed, and which the organization of the human body proclaims was meant to be attained by one and all of the members of the human family.

By avoiding the causes of disease which have been detailed in this work, and by attending to the rules which have been laid down here and elsewhere for the preservation of health, disease will be greatly abated, but a mighty revolution must be accomplished in the habits, the dispositions, and minds of men, ere mankind will enjoy that course of health, and all that greater freedom from pain and disease, of which their lot is capable:—but far from the consideration of the manifold changes and long course of time which will be required to make a very great improvement in the health of the human race, leading to apathy and inaction, it should serve to stimulate to powerful attempts, and persevering and reiterated efforts for amelioration.

THE END

www.ingramcontent.com/pod-product-compliance
Lightning Source LLC
LaVergne TN
LVHW022219200926
848481LV00006B/2037

9798348513320